RESHAPING DEMENTIA CARE

Practice and Policy in Long-Term Care

Miriam K. Aronson

editor

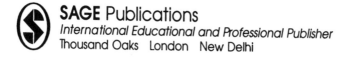

SAGE Publications
International Educational and Professional Publisher
Thousand Oaks London New Delhi

For information address:

SAGE Publications, Inc.
2455 Teller Road
Thousand Oaks, California 91320

SAGE Publications Ltd.
6 Bonhill Street
London EC2A 4PU
United Kingdom

SAGE Publications India Pvt. Ltd.
M-32 Market
Greater Kailash I
New Delhi 110 048 India

Printed in the United States of America

Library of Congress Cataloging-in-Publication Data

Main entry under title:

Reshaping dementia care : practice and policy in long-term care / edited by Miriam K. Aronson
    p. cm.
    Includes bibliographical references and index.
    ISBN 0-8039-5159-0 (cl). – ISBN 0-8039-5160-4 (pbk.)
    1. Senile dementia–Patients–Long-term care. 2. Senile dementia–Patients–Long-term care–United States. I. Aronson, Miriam K.
    [DNLM: 1. Dementia, Senile. 2. Long-Term Care–organization & administration–United States. 3. Long-Term Care–in old age. WT 150 R433 1994]
RC524.R47 1994
362.2'6–dc20
DNLM/DLC
                                     94-11316

94 95 96 97 10 9 8 7 6 5 4 3 2 1

Sage Production Editor: Diana E. Axelsen

Contents

Foreword

Reshaping Dementia Care:
Nursing Home Practice and Policy

Dementia in the elderly represents a serious public health problem because its prevalence is increasing, its impact upon affected individuals and families is high, and because at present there is no cure. Because of dementia's debilitating consequences nursing home care is frequently necessary. However, nursing home care is often viewed as a last resort or something akin to "giving up or giving in."

What is it about nursing homes that leads to these perceptions? Much of it emerges from their historical origins, namely the alms houses and mental institutions of the 19th century. This legacy is increasingly reinforced by the high prevalence of mental disorders, particularly dementia, in nursing homes and the limitations of psychiatric care in this setting. Fear and stigma associated with "losing one's mind" or one's dignity, or depending upon others for the most basic functions of life also are certainly frightening prospects. Most nursing homes have done little to challenge these perceptions by developing approaches to care that emphasize humanism, concern for individuals, and rehabilitation to enable individuals to achieve the fullest expression of their capacities. Consequently, improving care in nursing home represents one of the most important current challenges in clinical medicine.

To meet this challenge Dr. Aronson and her collaborators in *Reshaping Dementia Care: Nursing Home Practice and Policy* have assembled a practical and detailed guide for physicians, nurses, administrators, social workers, lawyers, families, and all others who seek to improve nursing home care in the United States today. The authors' teamwork and purpose convey the sense that this book was generated by friends and colleagues who have talked with one another and have agreed upon the important issues to be addressed. Each chapter illuminates a unique and relevant domain of nursing home care. The cumulative result is a substantial body of knowledge that guides us into advanced levels of thought, practice, and policy.

Particularly notable chapters include "Approaches to Special Programming" and "The Nursing Home Environment and Dementia Care" which describe inventive environmental adaptations and activity programs based upon the authors' extensive experience. "Reimbursement Issues and the Future Direction of Nursing Home Care for Persons With Dementia" provides a well-balanced discussion of the limitations of the current system of care for the elderly as well as suggestions for potential solutions. This book provides evidence that until existing programs are given flexibility by regulatory and reimbursement authorities to permit and encourage adaptation to evolving demands, barriers to access will continue to plague the system. Moreover, were the problem of access to be solved the problem of providing quality care would remain. Quality care must "take into account the way peoples' lives and their medical and psychosocial conditions are linked, so that what they need is available when they need it, in a way that respects their dignity and protects their rights" (p. 159, this volume).

People who are devoted to caring for persons with dementia will be better able to continue their care with energy, optimism, and confidence after reading this book. The nihilism and helplessness that pervades many nursing homes can be reshaped by the clear focus and guidance this work provides. Dr. Aronson's own empirical research, which informs much of what is written here, demonstrates the limitations of existing ways of conceptualizing and reimbursing nursing home care. Although she indicates that "the widespread availability of appropriate, competent, and adequately funded services is still more a dream than a reality" (pp. 41-42, this volume), *Reshaping Dementia Care* is a first step toward that reality for patients with dementia, their families, and their caregivers.

Barry W. Rovner, M.D.

Acknowledgments

There has been a dramatic increase in public awareness regarding Alzheimer's disease and other dementias during the last 15 years. Likewise, there has been a substantial heightening of research efforts to find causes, a cure, and ultimately prevention. Simultaneously, as a result of the increasing longevity of very old persons, there has been a marked increase in the number of afflicted individuals. Absent a cure, it is the ongoing care and management that is important for today's dementia victims. This book is designed for their caregivers.

I would like to acknowledge the extensive knowledge and commitment to excellence of the contributors, whose collective experience and enthusiasm will help to guide both professional and family caregivers in their important work.

I would like to thank the New York State Department of Health and specifically Dr. Mary Jane Koren, then Director of the Bureau of Long Term Care, for funding the projects and the 1991 conference upon which this book is based. None of this could have been accomplished without the administrative efforts of two of my colleagues, Dr. Donna Cox Post and Mr. Paul Guastadisegni, who were instrumental in making the conference and its proceedings a reality and who have contributed to individual chapters as well.

I must also recognize the conference Advisory Committee for their guidance and support; Arlene Barbera, R.N., C., B.S.N.; Joseph Breed, M.F.A., M.P.S., L.N.H.A.; Kenn Brown, L.N.H.A.; Cynthia Frazier, Ph.D.; Ralph Hall, M.A.; Jean Marks, M.Ed; Alan Morse, J.D., Ph.D.; Lila Sherlock, R.N., C., M.S.N.; Marc Sternberg, Ed.D; and Elaine Yatzkan, Ph.D.

I applaud the efforts of Karen Lazar for her assistance with manuscript preparation, and also Alucca Maraschini and Mary Bradshaw. Diana Axelsen, our Sage production editor, was most helpful.

Most of all, thank you to all the wonderful caregivers who tirelessly but silently provide life-sustaining services day in and day out. They are an ever-available source of information and expertise.

Miriam K. Aronson, Ed.D.

1

Overview of Dementia and the Nursing Home

Miriam K. Aronson

During the 20th century there has been unprecedented growth in the number and proportion of persons over 65 years of age in the population. In addition, there has been increased longevity for the oldest old, that is, those over 85. This trend is projected to continue with the increase in the number of the oldest old outstripping any other population subgroup. It has profound implications for the health and social policy of the nation, because the very old are the heaviest users of expensive health and long-term care services. With the escalating national debt and runaway health care costs, there is an outcry for health care reform and cost containment. Efforts in this regard must consider expenditures for long-term care, which now exceed $80 billion annually and are projected to triple within the next 30 years. Given the fact that dementia now accounts for more than half of nursing home admissions, dementia care is a high-priority issue.

Demographic Realities

Because of public health advances such as vaccination and treatment of infections, the average life expectancy is longer; hence, the proportion of elderly in the world's population continues to grow (Figure 1.1). For the United States, estimates are that the elderly, who currently make up 12.7% of the population, will represent 22% of the population by the year 2030. Although minority populations currently represent 13% of the elderly in this country, this proportion will double by 2030. The age distribution of the elderly is shown in Figure 1.2. The over-85 subgroup of elderly has grown over 60-fold from 1900-1990 (Figure 1.3); the growth will be even more dramatic in future years. The oldest old are the most at risk for nursing home placement.

Health Care Expenses

Older persons are heavier users of health services than those of other age groups. Although they comprised 12.7% of the population in 1987, they accounted for 36% of total personal health care expenditures. They accounted for 47% of all days of care in hospitals in 1991. Older persons averaged twice as many contacts with physicians than did persons under 65. Hospital expenditures accounted for 42% of older persons' health expenditures, followed by physicians (21%) and nursing home care (20%). Government benefits programs, including Medicare and Medicaid, covered about two thirds of health care expenditures by older persons. Fowles (1993).

Nursing Homes

On any given day, approximately 5% of persons over 65 reside in a nursing home, but the numbers rise dramatically

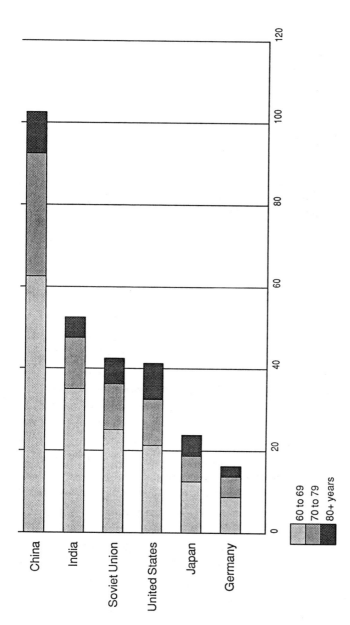

Figure 1.1. The World's Largest Elderly Populations Over Age 60–1991 (in millions)

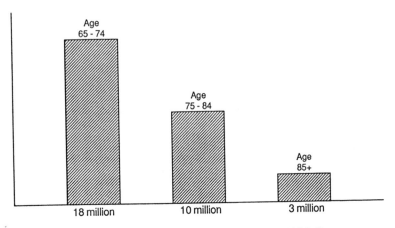

Figure 1.2. The United States Elderly Population—1990 Census
SOURCE: U.S. Bureau of the Census.
NOTE: *N* = 31.1 million.

with age—1% for persons 65-74; 6% for those 75-84; and 24% for those 85 and above. The number of elderly using a nursing home during the course of a year is much higher than the actual number of beds and is expected to increase dramatically. This is not a reflection of where the elderly prefer to receive chronic care; in fact, most would rather remain in their homes. Nevertheless, there are approximately 1.6 million nursing home beds in the United States. In 1985, 2.3 million elderly used a nursing home, and this figure is projected to be 4 million by the year 2018 (U.S. Accounting Office, Publication GAO/HRD). This growth makes the provision of nursing home care and other long-term care alternatives a pressing concern for society.

Payment for nursing home care comes predominantly from two sources: Medicaid, an entitlement program for "medically indigent" individuals that is funded jointly by the federal government and the government of each state, and private payment by individuals. Medicare, the federal program that is part of the Social Security system, pays for only a small proportion of

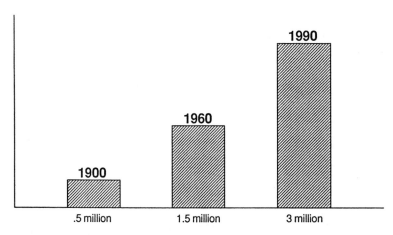

Figure 1.3. Growth of the 85+ Population
SOURCE: U.S. Bureau of the Census.

nursing home costs (less than 5%), and private long-term care insurance pays for even less.

Nursing Home Reform

The subject of nursing home care provided by nursing homes for vulnerable elderly has been fraught with episodic investigations and scandals. The attention given to nursing homes waxed and waned until 1986, when a report was issued by the Institute of Medicine entitled *Improving the Quality of Care in Nursing Homes.* This report described the widespread poor care in nursing homes and asserted the importance of quality of care and quality of life and the interrelationship between the two. The report became the basis for nursing home reform, which was embodied in the Omnibus Budget Reconciliation Act of 1987 (OBRA 87). Because regulation and enforcement are a combined effort of the federal government and the government of each state and because some of the recommendations will cost money to put into action, the total implementation of this legislation is incomplete; however, important inroads have been made.

OBRA 87 elevated the standards of care and had the following provisions and effects:

Residents' rights became an overriding consideration, affording each nursing home resident the opportunity to function at the "highest practicable level of mental and physical health."

Resident assessment was mandated, with the goal of obtaining current accurate information for individualized care planning. The Minimum Data Set (MDS) tool became the standard for accomplishing this.

Training and certification of nursing assistants were required to elevate the standards of practice of the nursing assistants, who are the primary hands-on caregivers in the nursing home, providing 90% of the direct care. Another important staffing provision was the mandated availability of sufficient professional staff, including social work and activities, to improve quality of life.

Preadmission screening and annual review (PASAAR) were introduced to assure that all nursing home applicants and residents in need of active mental health treatment were not "dumped" into nursing homes inappropriately.

Reduction of physical and chemical restraint use was mandated to assure that residents were not being restrained in place of receiving care. This was a most important provision for those with dementia, who account for the majority of "behavior problems" in the nursing home. Of equal importance was the fact that the very restraints that were being used for "safety purposes" were found to be detrimental to residents' function in terms of mobility, continence, and autonomy.

Establishment of a quality assurance committee was required to review goals and outcomes.

These OBRA 87 requirements have elevated the standards of care for all nursing home residents and have been most important in terms of care for the demented.

Dementing Illness

Dementing illness is the predominant cause of mental impairment among the elderly. Alzheimer's disease is the most common form of dementia, followed by multi-infarct (vascular) dementia and mixed Alzheimer's and vascular dementia. Prevalence increases markedly with advancing age: Although dementia affects less than 1% of persons aged 65, as many as one third to one half of persons aged 85 and over are afflicted. This high prevalence coincides with the period of life when individuals use health care services most heavily and are at great risk for needing nursing home and other long-term care services. The average age of admission to nursing homes is currently in the mid-80s. It is, therefore, no accident that the majority of nursing home residents are demented.

Dementia involves progressive declines in intellectual, functional, and behavioral abilities. Cognitive manifestations include memory loss, decrements in judgment, loss of ability to learn new things, perceptual difficulties, disorientation, loss of language skills, and changes in personality. These cognitive changes affect the capacity to survive independently, and afflicted individuals may eventually lose the ability to perform even the most routine activities of daily living. Associated behavioral symptoms, such as agitation, paranoia, depression, insomnia, and resistance to nursing care compound and confound each other and make some individuals more difficult to care for than others.

Behavioral Symptoms

Although dementia is an organic brain disease, many of its symptoms mimic psychiatric illness and are prevalent regardless of whether affected individuals reside at home or in institutions. Prevalence estimates of behavioral symptoms in nursing home patients range from 22.6% to 80%. This variability is due, in part, to classification issues. A recent analysis of data from the 1987 National Medical Expenditures Survey revealed a 53.5% prevalence rate of behavior problems in nursing home residents, with a not-so-different 44.3% prevalence among residents in personal care homes. There were a mean of 1.3 problem behaviors for nursing home residents and 0.9 for personal care residents. The most prevalent problem reported was getting upset/yelling. The study's authors delineated possible "biological, psychological, environmental and socio-cultural risk factors" for disruptive behaviors in institutional residents. (Jackson, Spector, & Rabins, 1993). Despite the high prevalence of behavioral symptoms in nursing homes, these facilities often have a dearth of mental health services.

Although approximately 4 million Americans currently have some form of dementia, it is estimated that by the year 2050, 14 million Americans will be afflicted. Alzheimer's disease was called the "Disease of the Century" in the 1980s by Dr. Lewis Thomas and will be the disease of two centuries as the 21st century approaches. Despite heightened biomedical research in the last decade or so and some promising leads, very little is known about the cause(s) of Alzheimer's disease or about effective pharmacologic treatment or prevention. Therefore, care of individuals with dementia will continue to be of great concern.

Families provide the bulk of necessary care in the home during most of the course of dementing illnesses. Despite the heroic efforts of many family caregivers, nursing home placement becomes a reality for some individuals. The factors that determine if and when a demented individual will be placed in a nursing home are not well delineated, nor are the predictors of what services will be needed once the individual is admitted. This is partially because demented individuals are themselves a heterogeneous group, differing according to severity of cognitive impairment, physical decline, associated behavior problems, and coexisting medical conditions.

Dementia and the Nursing Home

Although persons with dementia are the typical residents of nursing homes, often these patients and facilities are not a good match. Whereas there has been a fairly recent proliferation of "special care units," the care requirements of a demented population have not been adequately delineated (U.S. Office of Technology Assessment, Publication CTA-H-540, 1992). Discussions regarding whether there should be special units for demented residents are ongoing. Standards for special care units have not been adopted by most states, although the Joint Commission on Accreditation of Health Care Organizations (Oakbridge Terrace, Illinois) has developed its own. How dementia care is organized has been receiving increased attention from researchers and policymakers.

Special Care Units

Dementia-specific special care units are based on the concept of homogeneous groupings and generally target activities for ambulatory confused, wandering, and agitated residents. It is estimated that fewer than 20% of all facilities currently have special care units. These units vary widely because there is no empirical evidence supporting any single model. In addition, there are pragmatic problems. First, there is little or no reimbursement for special care units. Second, segregating one group of residents may not be practical for smaller facilities. It creates significant marketing problems: Finding a suitable applicant to fill a special care unit bed when one becomes available may not be immediately possible. Facilities without special units are able to avoid this economic snag and accept the next available applicant. Furthermore, residents develop increased needs as their disease progresses and may require transfer to another unit, which may not be available within the same facility. Thus, either a facility may need several special care units for patients with different severity of disease, or long-term patients may require transfers to other facilities. Ideally, quality care for residents with dementia would be available in every facility, with or without segregated units. Unfortunately, dementia know-how is not widespread, so this is not the case. Therefore, special care units currently have the potential to serve an important function as models of care and as training sites for the development of better dementia services.

Essentially, there has been little or no funding through traditional nursing home funding streams for the development of dementia services. This is partially attributable to a bias in the current reimbursement systems. The focus of long-term care payers is on paying for "skilled" nursing care—direct, hands-on interventions such as dressings, injections, and medical rehabilitation services. The needs of the demented are high-touch rather than high-tech interventions—mainly supervision, monitoring, direction, and cuing—and are not rewarded by the current system. This bias toward "heavier" care is also reflected in facility design. Although the nursing home is generally a facility for long-term residential chronic care, it is, in fact, designed, operated, and regulated like a hospital model. This is incongruous because nursing facilities are home to their residents for a substantial amount of time (an average of 2.5 years).

Determining Care Outcomes

An enormous challenge in developing dementia-specific services is evaluating their outcomes. Measurement of outcomes is difficult for the following reasons:

- Dementia involves a relentless biological progression for which there is no antidote, so that no matter how good the services are, the patients will ultimately exhibit declines in function.
- Dementia involves unpredictability and variability in behaviors and symptoms that are confounding to measure.
- There is no single biological marker that would enable confirmation of a diagnosis of Alzheimer's disease or quantification of level of disease in this long-term illness, so that patients are not easily comparable for purposes of measuring outcomes.
- Although certain interventions may seem positive empirically, there are no standard, accepted treatments that can be used as

a "gold standard," against which other interventions can be measured.

- Regulations and reimbursements are so variable throughout the country that obtaining comparability across states and facilities is difficult.
- Indications for nursing home placement are highly variable and are often a function of availability of social or financial supports and of available beds rather than severity of illness, adding yet another confound to the comparability issue.

Commensurate with all of these limitations is a lack of funding within the system for dementia-specific services (U.S. Office of Technology Assessment and U.S. Government Accounting Office).

Health Care Reform

Given the current political climate and public pressure to make health care more accessible and cost effective, it is likely that future care of the elderly will be modified. The emphasis will be shifted from the institution to the community. This will ultimately bring some chronic and long-term care services into the mainstream of health care. The focus will be on maintaining the frail elderly and disabled in their homes for as long as possible. Home care will be more accessible, and it is likely that financial subsidization for this will be available. Current reform proposals include broader eligibility criteria for services based on actual level of disability. Depending on how federal and state policies ultimately are developed, the expansion of home and community-based care will impact the availability of funding for nursing home services.

The Future of the Nursing Home

I predict that nursing homes will be utilized by the sickest and most dependent subset of the frail elderly once they can no longer be maintained at home. In all likelihood, the nursing home will become a subacute care facility, providing such services as ventilators, intensive rehabilitation, wound care, infusion therapies, and nutritional support. Nursing homes of the future will look more like the community hospitals of today, catering to sicker, less ambulatory patients who require more specialized, more technological medical interventions.

As the nursing home becomes more specialized and hospital-like, there will be need for the creative development of a range of services for older persons whose care needs are less intensive; hence, a whole new market for providers of geriatric care will open up. More for-profit entrepreneurs will enter this emerging market as there are more funds to spend on care, whether through governmental subsidy, private insurance, or personal means.

Care Options

An attractive option that can be a nursing home alternative for all but the bedfast individuals is that of "assisted living." Assisted living includes a broad spectrum of models such as foster care, board and care, residential care, boarding homes, congregate living with supervision and personal care services, and continuing care retirement communities.

Assisted living is less regulated than nursing homes and offers services to the frail elderly in a variety of formats. One format is to provide a service package that includes room and board, supervision, activities, and transportation to medical appointments. Personal care, nursing, and medical services are not included in this package and must be paid for as utilized. Thus, services that are now included in nursing home care are then "unbundled" into their component parts, which individuals can purchase according to their needs and pocketbooks. For example, some individuals may be able to manage their own medications, whereas others may require a nurse to do this. Nursing time can then be purchased, sometimes in increments as small as 15 minutes. Similarly, residents may need assistance with bathing, which may also be purchased. Thus, this type of residential care is less costly because services are provided only to those who need them.

Certain groups have found assisted living to be an attractive format for developing dementia-specific facilities because there are opportunities for experimentation with new models of care. It is conceivable that special care dementia units of the future will become a feature of assisted living rather than nursing homes. Assisted living offers the opportunity for innovative architectural design. It also provides for more flexible staffing, for example, cross-trained personal care aides who perform multidisciplinary functions such as personal care, activities, and meal service. Assisted living generally has fewer licensed personnel than nursing homes. For example, a facility may have only one consulting registered nurse, rather than a nursing department. Residents use their own physicians so there is not necessarily a staff physician. The ability to devise less medicalized services for the ambulatory confused is appealing because the emphasis can be placed on other aspects of care. However, there is a caveat: Although individuals with dementia may require less medicalized services, they do not necessarily require less care.

The opportunities for innovation in assisted living are exciting; yet the latitude given providers can be a boon to the unscrupulous. Somehow a middle ground must be found so that appropriate quality services can be developed.

Funding

With the exception of Oregon, where residential options have been incorporated into the long-term care reimbursement system, assisted living facilities are either paid for privately or by very limited social security/social service funding. The result is a variety of facilities that range from marginal to luxurious. Until the policymakers acknowledge that people prefer some type of assisted living rather than nursing home care and, accordingly, make funds available, this option will not develop to its full potential.

The Challenge

The challenge to care providers is to devise a range of services for people with the same condition, that is, dementia, but with differing constellations of symptoms that change as the disease progresses. Appropriate dementia care, both in the community and within the nursing home, thus requires a continuum of services, whose configuration is as yet emerging. Two areas of extreme importance in this regard are provider and consumer training and education.

References

Fowles, D. G. (1993). *A profile of older Americans.* Washington, DC: American Association of Retired Persons.

Jackson, E., Spector, W., & Rabins, P. (1993). Risk of behavior problems among U.S. nursing and personal care home residents. *Gerontologist, 33* (1), 193.

Long term care: projected needs of the aging baby boom generation (Report GAO/HRD 91-86). Washington, DC: U.S. Government Accounting Office.

U.S. Congress, Office of Technology Assessment. (1992, August). *Special care units for people with Alzheimer's and other dementias: consumer education, research, regulatory and reimbursement issues* (Report OTA-H-540). Washington, DC: Government Printing Office.

2

Current Challenges
in Dementia Care

A Physician's Perspective

Leonard Berg

Despite important advances in understanding the causes of dementia and developing new potential treatments, it is clear that answers to the major questions of causes, prevention, and cures will not be available until some years from now. Because society is aging and the prevalence of dementia rises with advancing age, the problems engendered by dementia will be increasing for the foreseeable future.

The challenges in dementia care are to meet goals despite the obstacles in the path. All agree that appropriate goals in caring for people with dementia include maintaining an optimal level of function and enhancing the quality of life at each stage of the illness. The standards for setting those goals should be in accord with ethical practice and with the explicit or perceived wishes of the individual who is demented. Examples of the obstacles found in long-term care institutions are all too familiar: rising costs of institutional care, fiscal constraints in reimbursement, the burden of providing heavy care for those who need it, and staff burnout.

Of the approximately 1.5 million residents of nursing homes in the United States, more than half are demented. Dementia has become the principal reason for admission to long-term care institutions and the major issue in maintaining appropriate programs. It is now well known that the principal cause of dementia is Alzheimer's disease (AD), not only in long-term care institutions but throughout the community. To the extent that appropriate methods are developed to improve care for people with AD, these issues will be largely addressed for all who are demented. The problems are increasing. A recent relevant publication of the U.S. Congress was entitled "Losing a Million Minds," but current estimates are that as many as 4 million people in this country suffer from AD. If current trends continue for the next 40 years, there will be 11 or 12 million people who are demented, most of whom have AD. Consider the problems of coping with three times as many demented people, finding the staff, finding the resources, building the residential facilities, and developing and maintaining a range of programs to support optimal function and enhance quality of life. These are already enormous challenges that will increase sharply over the next few decades.

What Is Dementia?

This symptom complex is defined as an overall deterioration of intellectual function in a fully awake person. Foremost is deterioration of memory, mainly for recent events, but eventually there is loss of memory even for events of years ago. Loss of orientation occurs, that is, an inability to find one's way even in familiar places and to keep track of what year and month it is. There is also deterioration of judgment, so that one's reasoning, the ability to evaluate conditions and make appropriate responses, is poor. In addition, dementia impairs language function and the ability to recognize spatial relationships or visual objects. Often there is a change in personality, sometimes an exaggeration of previous personality traits, sometimes a reversal of traits, sometimes a total loss of personality, the features that made the person a unique, recognizable individual. That change in personality may be the manifestation most troubling to the family as they watch their relative deteriorate. Finally, dementia leads to loss of ability to perform even the most routine activities of daily living.

Definition and Diagnosis of Alzheimer's Disease

Dementia is caused most often by Alzheimer's disease, not "senility . . . just old age . . . hardening of the arteries . . . little strokes." Alzheimer's disease is a brain disease accompanied by characteristic microscopic structural changes in brain tissue by which its presence can be proved at autopsy. These features of AD are neurofibrillary tangles that are coarse strands of abnormal protein filaments within nerve cells and senile plaques, composed of globular deposits of another abnormal protein called amyloid with an admixture of degenerating nerve cell endings.

Even though proof of AD requires microscopic examination of brain tissue by biopsy or autopsy, experienced physicians are quite accurate in making the diagnosis based only on clinical evidence. Dementia is diagnosed by recognizing the characteristic global impairment of intellectual function in an alert individual. The differential diagnosis, that is, the determination of the cause of the dementia, requires a full history, appropriate examinations, and the results of certain laboratory tests. Obtaining the history of the onset and course of the disorder from someone who knows the person well is critical. A stable dementia with abrupt onset may result from an acute head injury, cardiac arrest that deprives the brain of its blood and oxygen supply, or prolonged severe hypoglycemia, as in an "insulin reaction" in a person with diabetes mellitus. Sometimes dementia results acutely from a subarachnoid hemorrhage or another type of stroke that results in death of critical parts of the brain necessary for normal intellectual function.

Far more frequently, dementia begins gradually, and its onset is difficult to date even by persons who know the individual well. In AD that gradual onset and progression are characteristic. There are no acute events in the early stages to suggest sudden insults to the brain, as by strokes. The condition gradually grows worse, even though there may be "good and bad days" or modest fluctuations in the level of dementia around an underlying course of steady decline. In the most clear-cut examples of AD there are no other major medical, neurologic, or psychiatric disorders that might be influencing a person's mental state. When these other disorders are significant factors, they can usually be recognized from a detailed medical history. Inquiring about exposure to medication is critical because of the frequency with which medication usage or its withdrawal can influence mental function.

Next, it is necessary to perform a complete general physical, neurologic, and psychiatric examination of the individual in order to detect signs of major systemic medical disease or important neurologic or psychiatric illness, such as Parkinson's disease, focal results of stroke, or major depression. The intellectual impairment is documented by a mental status examination that includes assessment of memory, orientation, language, ability to calculate, judgment, and mood. Several standardized brief questionnaires are available to test those components of the mental state. Examples are the Mini-Mental State Exam of Folstein and colleagues and Pfeiffer's Short Portable Mental Status Questionnaire. Formal psychometric testing is rarely necessary for making a diagnosis.

Because some specific causes of dementia may not offer clues to their presence in the history or examination, it is appropriate to include a short list of laboratory tests as a relatively standardized battery. The following are usually recommended: complete blood count, blood chemistry profile, serology for syphilis and HIV infection when appropriate, serum vitamin B-12 level, thyroid function tests, and an imaging

TABLE 2.1 Disorders to Be Considered in Differential Diagnosis of AD

A. Medical (e.g., drug toxicity, hypothyroidism, kidney or liver failure, vitamin B-12 deficiency)

B. Psychiatric (e.g., major depression)

C. Degenerative brain diseases (e.g., Parkinson's, Pick's, Huntington's diseases)

D. Other brain diseases (e.g., multiple infarcts or strokes, brain tumor, hydrocephalus, subdural hematoma, HIV infection, neurosyphilis, multiple sclerosis)

study of the brain. When the history indicates chronic dementia, a noncontrast computed tomographic (CT) scan is usually sufficient. Only rarely is the extra information from CT contrast material or magnetic resonance imaging (MRI) needed, and both of these procedures add to the expense of investigation. Similarly, electroencephalographic (EEG) or spinal fluid examinations are rarely indicated in the differential diagnosis of AD. Other expensive tests, such as evoked potentials and emission tomography (SPECT or PET), are sometimes recommended by enthusiasts or entrepreneurs, but thus far these tests have not been shown to perform as well as the judgment of an experienced physician, and they rarely add anything valuable to differential diagnosis. Note that there is no specific laboratory test that establishes the diagnosis of AD; the tests are used to rule out other disorders that may mimic AD (Table 2.1). If the clinical diagnosis is made according to appropriate standards, the diagnosis of AD will be confirmed by autopsy in close to 90% of patients.

Behavioral Disorders

Dementia may give rise to troublesome behaviors, mood disorders, and psychotic manifestations that complicate the problems of dealing with the intellectual impairment. These behavioral disorders are frequent in persons whose dementia is more than mild. Some of these phenomena are agitation, assault/aggression (actual or threatened), wandering, screaming, and depression/apathy/withdrawal. Sleep disorders and inappropriate sexual behaviors may create problems. Agitated persons with dementia often show psychotic manifestations such as delusions and hallucinations. It is important to remember that agitation may result from some unrecognized source of pain, for instance, an undiagnosed fracture, because the dementia prevents the person from telling others about the pain. Behavioral disorders are a primary source of stress for families and are often the major reason for institutionalization.

Both pharmacologic and nonpharmacologic treatments for these manifestations are to be considered after evaluating the situation in an effort to identify and eliminate the precipitating factors. There have been many suggestions that effectiveness can be demonstrated both for behavioral methods and various pharmacologic agents. However, most of these reports are anecdotal rather than based on controlled studies. There are some promising nonpharmacologic approaches to the treatment of agitation. These include reassuring physical contact, use of pet animals, behavior modification techniques, and simple oral communication. Music therapy may be useful.

In general, drugs should be reserved until nondrug approaches have been shown to be unsuccessful. The side effects of medication for these disorders include oversedation, shuffling, falling, and difficulty swallowing. Drugs may paradoxically increase agitation or depression. Nevertheless, there appears to be a place for the properly monitored use of antidepressants, tranquilizers, and antipsychotic agents. However, the automatic prescription of tranquilizers in response to a disturbing behavior is to be deplored.

What is needed is systematic research by multiple groups of investigators in order to establish the effectiveness of various treatments. Attention must be paid to rigorous definition of the symptoms under investigation, development of research instruments with which to measure the frequency and severity of the behavioral disorders, and proper design of controlled studies to evaluate pharmacologic and nonpharmacologic interventions.

Families and the Burden of Care

It is remarkable how family caregivers carry on despite the enormous burdens—physical, emotional, financial—of caring for their loved ones who have AD. When Jack Pollack, the Brooklyn high school principal, and his wife were pictured on the cover of *Newsweek,* she already had had AD for about 10 years. She was completely helpless and no longer spoke. Even so, he was maintaining her at home, as is true of most families dealing with AD. In addition to his full-time employment, he was caring for his wife at night and on the weekends, while during the workday he had hired help for her care.

How do families manage? Help is available from the Alzheimer's Association in the form of education, support, and advice. Day-care centers and other forms of respite care can relieve some of the caregiver burden on family caregivers. Families, volunteers, and health professionals work together to keep these impaired people with dementia out of institutions.

Designing Programs of Care

The goals of care for people with dementia, in or out of institutions, are to maintain optimal levels of function as long as possible and to maintain or enhance the quality of life. The needs of the resident should remain the focus of attention in designing the package of care modalities to help reach these goals. In long-term care institutions the package includes the physical and emotional environment, staff, programming, and appropriate input from the family.

The environment. A large and crowded dining room frequently adds to the confusion of residents with dementia. Smaller areas with less bustle seem to work better. Lighting, cuing, signage, noise control, and wandering areas can be helpful. Remember that wandering is a problem for the staff or family caregivers, not for the individual with dementia. When one provides a secure inside or outside area for walking, wandering, or exercise, one usually reduces the level of agitation and the need for considering restraints. Environment can be used to advantage when designed with the needs of the demented individual in mind.

Staffing. It is important to recruit and select appropriate caring people to work in long-term care, to implement appropriate training procedures, and to provide professional development for staff. Important responsibilities of administrators are to attend to the emotional and physical needs of staff, to help keep them efficient and effective, to avoid staff burnout, and to minimize staff turnover.

Programming. Planning a care program includes the use of an interdisciplinary team. Ideally, staff meet to develop an individual plan of care appropriate for the person with dementia. The care plan should be based on an understanding of the interests and strengths of that person before he or she became demented as well as a thorough appraisal of his or her current status.

Many long-term care activities programs appropriate for nondemented residents work poorly for the demented. However, certain activities, such as gardening, cleaning, or simple kitchen tasks, are often useful. Special programs for the individual with dementia may include music. Its almost universal appeal means that singing and dancing will be appropriate long after the ability to carry on a reasonable conversation is lost. Innovative approaches and the integration of environment, staffing, and programming will help reach those goals of maintaining optimal function and quality of life. Teenage volunteers may work well in helping residents with their activities.

The family. Although most family caregivers remain interested in their relatives, not all families are able or willing to continue to be involved after placement in a nursing home. When they are willing, they can help with feeding and activity programs and thus can relieve some of the burden on staff.

Changes in Residents Over Time
(Progression, Delirium, Depression)

Dementia in AD is not a static disorder. It worsens over time, and the individual's level of function declines. Modifications in staff expectations and in the resident's care plan will be needed. However, keep in mind that AD does not lead to abrupt declines in mental function. When a resident with AD suddenly becomes worse, one must realize that something else has been added to the clinical picture of AD. The complication is often a delirium that may be corrected by appropriate treatment. *Delirium* is an acute mental disorder characterized by decreased awareness of the environment and difficulty maintaining proper attention to people and objects nearby. The name is derived from a Latin term meaning "off the track." Other terms that are used to refer to the same disorder include acute confusional state, acute brain syndrome, and acute metabolic encephalopathy. The inattentiveness and decreased awareness lead to mental confusion. Persons in this state of delirium may be quiet and drowsy, or they may be agitated, noisy, restless, and hostile. Their speech is often incomplete and slurred or mumbling. Misinterpretations, delusions, and hallucinations are common. The abnormal mental state often fluctuates in delirium and may be accompanied by rapid heart rate, fluctuating blood pressure, and episodes of sweating and flushed appearance.

Older individuals are much more susceptible to delirium than younger adults and may become acutely confused even when their baseline mental status is perfectly normal. A very long list of acute diffuse insults to the brain may cause delirium, including fever, infection, dysfunction of many organ systems, disturbance in blood chemistry, and the effects of medication or its withdrawal. Anesthesia often makes an older person susceptible to delirium.

Another important cause of deterioration in AD is *depression*. One must maintain a high level of suspicion that depression may be present because it can cause major deterioration of function in dementia, just as it may cause profound impairment of function in the person who is not demented. Some of the symptoms of depression may mimic or overlap those of dementia. To further complicate the picture, depression often coexists with dementia, especially early in the course. Appropriate drug therapy will usually reverse the effects of depression.

Need for Continuous Assessment/Reassessment

These are some of the reasons why it is critically important not only to evaluate persons with dementia fully before the original care plan is designed, but to reevaluate their condition and needs periodically to determine whether another factor has intervened and should be addressed. Persons with dementia are at increased risk of falling and of having medication reactions, for example. The watchword should be constantly evaluating people with dementia, addressing their needs, determining what has caused a recent deterioration of function, and providing appropriate treatment.

Special Care Programs and Units

Special care units for dementia or AD patients have been proliferating for about 10 years. Even though many health professionals feel confident from their own experience that special programs have been beneficial, it has not yet been possible to prove that conclusion by rigorous research methods. With all of the variables to be considered, such as characteristics of residents, families, staff members, programs, and physical environments, it has been difficult to carry out well-designed and well-controlled experimental studies to answer the questions of whether changes in environment or staff training, for instance, have a significant beneficial impact on residents with dementia.

Nevertheless, researchers and practitioners have been comparing notes and collaborating to devise better ways to conduct these experiments. One hopes that the next few years will provide answers relevant to the best ways to care for people with dementia, whether at home or in institutions.

Segregation Versus Integration of Residents With Dementia

This issue is related to the question of the role of special care units. Among the factors in favor of segregation of residents with dementia is their need for security, dignified personal care, and protection from exploitation or abuse. Furthermore, nondemented but frail residents are entitled to privacy, choice, and an environment safe from disruptions and invasions by intrusive, inappropriate, and often impulsive residents with dementia. Some professionals, however, believe that the potential gains resulting from clustering residents with dementia in a segregated unit are counterbalanced by negative features such as the stigma associated with segregation and the absence of nondemented individuals as role models with whom demented individuals may interact.

Obstacles to Reaching Goals

Governmental regulations, such as those related to the Omnibus Budget Reconciliation Act (OBRA), clearly are beneficial by intent. They speak to the important issues of residents' rights and the inappropriate use of restraints, whether pharmacologic or mechanical. However, it has been difficult for professionals in the industry to adapt to the ever-changing regulations. The "small print" attached thereto is frequently difficult to interpret and apply. Regulations may inhibit the development of special care programs, especially when requirements change from year to year. Nevertheless, the unshackling of many residents of nursing homes that has resulted clearly has improved the quality of life for some residents with dementia. In some facilities individuals are still restrained excessively and inappropriately; abuses persist. The current case-mix reimbursement system adds to the problems by not recognizing the extra costs inherent in caring for those with dementia.

A serious problem for caregivers, whether family members or paid caregivers, is the prevalence of behavioral disorders that may appear during the course of dementia. There are the repetitive questions that result from severe memory loss ("Where's my mother?" "Where are we going today?"). Thirty seconds after one has dealt with the question, it is repeated. These incessant questions may be very burdensome, because they reflect not only the loss of memory but also the insecurity and agitation that appear in the dementia syndrome.

Other behavioral problems include an excessive emotional response ("catastrophic reaction") to minor disturbances in the environment and the paranoid thinking that leads to suspiciousness and repetitious accusations ("I can't find my purse; you must have taken it."). The demented person does not consider the possibility that he or she has misplaced belongings but is likely to accuse others of having taken them.

Also contributing to staff burnout in long-term care institutions is the increased numbers of residents who have multiple disorders and require intensified nursing and medical care. Many require maximum help from staff for survival—complete care in bathing, dressing, feeding, toileting, positioning—a constant responsibility.

The Financial Crunch

The increasing costs of health care, whether inside or out of institutions, come at a time when fiscal crises are occurring everywhere. As government bodies (national, state, local) have more difficulty meeting their financial obligations, society must deal with the costs of care for the current 1.5 million residents of nursing homes across the country and contemplate the increased numbers expected over the next few decades.

Many are hopeful there will be a change in national policy toward long-term care, whether by a government-pay program or by a combined government and private insurance initiative. However, a fundamental change in the system over the next few years is unlikely. Congress was badly burned a few years ago in its attempt to address a related problem, when it passed the catastrophic health care bill to deal with the financial problems of care for the elderly.

Families preparing for institutionalization commonly conclude they should distribute the assets of the person with dementia in order that the person qualify for Medicaid. Books provide advice on how to protect life savings by placing assets in trust or dividing them among relatives in order to "spend down" quickly and qualify for Medicaid. It is curious that the same individuals who matured with the attitude that one should save to care for one's needs in old age are being encouraged not to "waste" those savings on caring for themselves, but rather to pass their assets on to children or other relatives and to let taxpayers foot the bill for institutional care. Given the constraints of national and local budget priorities and capacities, it may not be realistic to expect taxpayers to shoulder the rapidly increasing costs of long-term care.

Ethical Issues

There are several guidelines appropriate for health care professionals dealing with institutional residents and patients with dementia elsewhere. The first principle, preserving life, has progressively evolved to include preserving the dignity or quality of life when one is dealing with advanced dementia. Two other long-standing principles are the admonishments to "do good" and "do no harm." In applying these guidelines it is appropriate to respect the fourth principle, patient autonomy, that is, the right of the individual to consider the likely benefits and burdens of a proposed treatment and to make choices concerning his or her care. At any point in the course of dementia, as long as an individual is able to participate intellectually in the decisions, it is that person's right to decide whether to accept or reject medical treatment.

The next principle has to do with acting with integrity. That means being honest with patients and their families—honest about realistic expectations and the consequences of a new plan of treatment. For instance, what can one expect if a person with far-advanced dementia develops life-threatening pneumonia? Acting with integrity means making it clear that curing the pneumonia will not lead to improvement in the underlying dementia. If anything, the additional trauma of serious pneumonia will have a lasting adverse impact, leaving the person more impaired than before the infection. Risks of aspiration will continue and lead to recurrent cycles of pneumonia, antibiotics, worsening of the dementia, more aspiration, and pneumonia again.

In the discussion of probable outcomes of a proposed therapy, families should know what to expect if the demented person's life is saved. Next there should be discussion of what the person with dementia would have wanted. That is, if the person were able to understand the issues, would he or she have said, "Treat my pneumonia and preserve my life even at this very low level of function," or would the request have been "Please keep me comfortable and let me die peacefully from the pneumonia"?

These are very difficult issues for almost everyone; yet they are important and must be addressed. The U.S. Supreme Court decided that each person has the right to die by rejecting treatment. However, the Court left it to the individual states to set the guidelines for how to determine whether a person who can no longer participate in the decision would want to refuse treatment. That is the reason to attend to the issue of advance directives with respect to autonomy. Everyone should encourage friends, relatives, patients, and residents to prepare living wills now, lest they become incapacitated before executing such a document. Living wills and the appointment of proxies for health care decisions should be put in place much more frequently than they are at present.

In the absence of written advance directives, who will make decisions concerning when a demented person should receive treatment and when treatment should be withheld or withdrawn? Most would answer that it should be the person who knows the demented individual best, a family member or close friend who knew that person before the dementia intervened. Studies suggest that relatives and friends who know the individual well are in a better position to predict what treatment the person would choose than are physicians, nurses, or social workers.

It is desirable to avoid involving the courts in making decisions on treatment issues. Family caregivers are appropriate surrogate decision makers. In each instance, one should consider the likely benefits and the likely harm or burden of that treatment. The phrase "benefit versus burden" is based on the two principles of "do good" and "do no harm." The benefits and burdens of treatment should be considered with respect to each level of medical and nursing care to be provided in the presence of advanced dementia. Should all modern technology available be applied, such as ventilators, intensive care units, transplant surgery? Should medications be used to sustain life or treat intercurrent infections? Should hydration and nutrition be continued by feeding tube when the person can no longer swallow? The answers to those questions should be based on the issue of benefit versus burden in the value system of the individual affected.

One level of treatment is never to be abandoned. The person's comfort, hygiene, and dignity must be maintained even when all other forms of treatment are withheld or withdrawn.

These are the ethical guidelines to be considered, with emphasis on the patient's autonomy, the right of the resident to make decisions on accepting or refusing treatment. When the person is no longer able to make those decisions, close family members or friends must use their own best judgment as surrogate decision makers, guided, one hopes, by evidence in written documents, such as a living will.

Conclusion

The current challenges in the care of people with dementia are to meet goals of maintaining an optimal level of their function and enhancing the quality of their lives, despite the obstacles of regulations that are sometimes inappropriate, budget constraints, and both physical and emotional burdens on family and staff caregivers. Those who work in this endeavor do so because of the satisfaction in caring for people who need help, not only the individual residents, but also their relatives, who are caught up in the enormous problems posed by dementia.

Suggested Readings

Berg, L, Buckwalter, L. D., Chafetz, P. K., et al. (1991). Special care units for persons with dementia. *Journal of the American Geriatrics Society, 39,* 1229-1236.

Cummings, J. L., & Miller, B. L. (Eds.). (1990). *Alzheimer's disease: Treatment and long-term management.* New York: Marcel Dekker.

Katzman, R. (1989). Delirium and dementia. In L. P. Rowland (Ed.), *Merritt's textbook of neurology* (8th ed., pp. 3-9). Philadelphia: Lea & Febiger.

Mace, N. L., & Rabins, P. V. (1991). *The 36-hour day* (rev. ed.). Baltimore, MD: Johns Hopkins University Press.

Ruark, J. E., Raffin, T. A., & Stanford University Medical Center Committee on Ethics. (1988). Initiating and withdrawing life support. *New England Journal of Medicine, 318,* 25-30.

Teri, L., Rabins, P., Whitehouse, P., Berg, L., Reisberg, B., Sunderland, T., Eichelman, B., & Phelps, C. (1993). Management of behavior disturbance in Alzheimer's disease: Current knowledge and future directions. *Alzheimer's Disease and Associated Disorders, 6*(2), 77-88.

Wragg, R. E., & Jeste, D. V. (1988). Neuroleptics and alternative treatments: Management of behavioral symptoms and psychosis in Alzheimer's disease and related conditions. *Psychiatric Clinics of North America, 11,* 195-213.

3

Dementia Care

Program and Staff Variables

Miriam K. Aronson

Dementia care is complex and requires a well-defined facility philosophy, commensurate program objectives, and policies and procedures for implementation. Dementia care requires adaptations of the environment and of staffing patterns, and ongoing training and support. In this chapter, care principles are discussed in relation to nursing home care, but they may be extrapolated to other settings as well.

Program Objectives

The basic objectives for care of nursing home residents are to know the resident, to assure the resident's physical safety and psychological security, and to encourage his or her functioning at the best possible level. In addition, residents need to have as much autonomy and control as possible, as well as socialization both within and outside the facility. Demented individuals need maximal environmental awareness and an appropriate amount of stimulation. Further, it is necessary to develop procedures and programs that are adaptable to changing and fluctuating needs.

Assessment

There is no substitute for thorough and continuous assessment of residents for development of appropriate, individualized care plans. Diagnoses are simply not enough. Even after a complete workup for dementia and the availability of a diagnosis, clinical personnel need additional information for care planning, including:

- *Ambulation status:* Is the individual ambulatory, chairfast, or bedfast? If ambulatory, does the patient have a history of leaving the unit or building without the knowledge of staff members?
- *Communication ability:* What are the verbal abilities? If there are expressive problems, how does the patient make her or his needs known? How much does he or she understand?
- *Activities of daily living:* Can the patient dress himself or herself? If not independently, could the patient do so with supervision and/or cuing? Can the patient eat independently? If not totally independently, could the patient substantially self-feed with modifications of diet such as finger foods?
- *Socialization:* Is the patient withdrawn or very active? What social skills does the individual have? Does he or she do better in group activities or in one-on-one situations? Does this person respond especially well to a particular staff person or approach?
- *Sleep pattern:* Sleep patterns need to be determined. Is the person an early riser? Is he or she accustomed to napping during the day? How many hours does he or she usually sleep?
- *Behavioral sequelae:* Do behavioral problems occur at a certain time of day, for example, in the late afternoon or early evening (i.e., sundowning)? Do behavioral problems occur in relation to certain situations (precipitants) such as bathing? Are these symptoms responsive to particular interventions?

- *Personality:* What are the individual's strengths? Major deficits? Which personality traits significantly affect care? For example, is the person basically a loner or a social individual? Is he or she stubborn or fairly flexible? What personality changes have occurred?

Assessment must be a dynamic, ongoing process, whereby changes are recognized and incorporated into individualized plans of care. This is a foundation for good care and is also mandated by provisions of the Omnibus Budget Reconciliation Act (OBRA).

Assuring Physical Safety

Environment is not a substitute for good care, but it is an important adjunct. Ideally, it should enable patient functioning. In many cases, however, the environment may be in conflict with basic program objectives. For example, long, poorly lit corridors can increase the confusion of already-confused residents, and confined spaces can make already-agitated wanderers more agitated. Lighting levels and furniture arrangement can contribute to safety.Increased confusion and/or agitation may contribute to accidents and incidents in residents whose judgment, orientation, and perception are compromised.

Simplification of the environment and prevention of clutter are adjuncts that will facilitate safe movement, as will control of the traffic pattern of other residents and staff. Access to a dementia unit should be limited. It should not be an area that staff walk through to get somewhere else. Entrances and exits to a dementia unit may need to be secured to promote easy movement within the unit, while preventing residents from leaving the area without authorization. Securing doorways is important, but no matter how sophisticated the alarm system, this is but one small facet of a dementia program.

Allowing residents to wander freely has been described as "therapeutic risk taking." Although the actual number of falls may be greater for demented than for nondemented residents, there is no increased significant injury. Walking may actually be helpful in preventing deconditioning and other problems associated with immobility. This information underlies the OBRA mandates regarding reduction of physical and chemical restraint use.

Enhancing Psychological Security

Hallmarks of dementia are confusion, loss of orientation, and loss of a sense of mastery. Thus, environments need to be infused with cues so that residents feel comfortable and familiar.

A key adaptation is creating spaces that are manageable for cognitively impaired residents, for example, by dividing larger units into smaller groupings. This can be accomplished by building design or, when this is not possible, by creative arrangement of furnishings. Having several small groups in a 40-bed unit, each with its own lounge, or at least sitting area, is preferable to long and undistinguished corridors with one large dayroom. Moving around smaller, intimate spaces can be more manageable for disoriented individuals.

Cues can be provided by personalization of the facility with familiar furnishings and objects—a favorite chair or piece of furniture, family pictures, or other memorabilia which make the surroundings more homelike. Instructional signs with both pictures and words can be helpful. Lighting, colors, and textures can provide cues that serve to track residents either toward or away from certain areas.

Autonomy and Control

Autonomy and control are especially important to individuals who are experiencing cognitive decline and feel that they are "losing it." Design and program elements may assist in providing opportunities for exercising control. For example, feelings of autonomy may be enhanced by openness and accessibility—openness to the outside, windows on busy areas such as the lobby and the street, accessibility from one area to another, as from the inside to an outdoor area or in and out of some interesting nooks and crannies. With defined boundaries there is less uncertainty and more opportunity for success. Feelings of control are also derived from having choices and structured opportunities for accomplishment, such as through modified activities programs.

Privacy

Privacy is a difficult goal to achieve in a nursing home, where shared bedrooms are the norm. Design elements can assist with this situation, however. Varying arrangements of furnishings can promote a sense of privacy, for example, toe-to-toe bed arrangements or the use of smaller private rooms off a common anteroom, rather than a larger shared bedroom. Storage and tracking of personal items are another privacy issue. Locked storage areas are difficult to administer because demented individuals may lose their keys or may not have the coordination or cognition to use them.

Promoting Socialization

Persons with dementia usually maintain good social skills despite their cognitive and functional declines, and socialization is an important program element. Social interaction can be promoted by the easy accessibility of public areas. For example, rooms facing a central garden or atrium allow for a resident to be a participant-observer of the action. Central, open nurses' stations allow for adequate work space with maintenance of interaction with residents. Availability of a warm and welcoming space for visitation encourages socialization, as do certain dining arrangements, such as smaller tables and permanent table mates. Also, the use of volunteers and community groups encourages the maintenance of connections with persons out-side the facility.

Adapting to Changing Needs

During the progressive course of dementia, the residents change, but their disease renders them unable to learn new things. Thus, rather than the residents adapting, it is the facility and staff that must do so. This involves having the space and the equipment to care for residents as they become more confused and less physically able. Bathing, toileting, and feed-ing activities will require adaptations. A good motto for staff working with demented individuals is "go with the flow." The program must be based on resident needs.

Maintaining Environmental Awareness

Interesting colors and textures, adequate lighting, appropri-ate sound levels, and creative arrangement of space are integral to maintaining environmental awareness. Special features may be included in specialized units but are not sufficient in and of themselves. Rather, they are adjunctive to appropriate staffing, staff training, a well-conceived program, and clinical expertise. Many facilities have incorporated the heavy use of props and memorabilia in a "memory lane" as a key component of their dementia program. These displays may be quite elaborate; however, they may sometimes impact the families of resident more than the residents themselves. As with other interven-tions, moderation is the key.

Because demented individuals may have language difficul-ties, multisensory cues may enhance remaining functional abili-ties. For example, pictures and words are more effective than words alone on signs identifying the toilet, the dining room, the telephone, or the resident's own room. Conversely, be-cause judgment and orientation are impaired, the camouflage of doors or door knobs may be helpful in discouraging residents from using them.

Controlling Stimulation

A good practice in dealing with individuals with dementia is to limit extraneous stimuli. Consider, for example, a paging system. Is such a system necessary on a dementia unit where residents may misinterpret the cues? Also, residents and staff benefit from a traffic pattern that is efficient and keeps unnecessary noise and distractions to a minimum. Although some residents need a low-stimulus setting, others may require more stimulation. The availability of multiple public areas may help in this regard. A high-stimulus activity such as dancing or exercise may be happening in one area, while residents are listening to soft music in another. Making sure the television is turned off in the dayroom while an activity is being conducted is another practice that can help residents focus their attention.

Staffing

There is no substitute for having enough competent staff members to provide good care; however, although having more staff may contribute to better care, it does not guarantee it. Multiple factors need to be considered. First, there is a need for adequate staffing. In addition to the ratio of staff to residents, the quality of the staff, the continuity, and the scheduling are important. Consideration must also be given to the ratio of professionals to paraprofessionals (nurses to nursing assistants in a given situation) and the presence of other health professionals, including activities, occupational therapy, physical therapy, and social service personnel. Are the numbers and types of staff readjusted with changes in case-mix? Are volunteers and families used to enhance the quality of life?

Continuity includes the stability and attendance of the staff. Two agency nurses on a shift may not be equal to one experienced regular employee. Staff rotation may disrupt the fragile stability of a confused resident who barely knows his or her caregivers. A primary care nursing model in which the same staff care for the same residents is helpful. Scheduling also impacts the operations of a unit. For example, enough staff need to be present during times of heavy activity, such as morning care and mealtimes.

The quality of the staff depends on how they are selected and trained. Selection involves choosing those most likely to succeed in working with difficult residents. Training is an essential ongoing activity and is discussed in a later section. Furthermore, job descriptions should be realistic and well conceived. Tasks must be analyzed for their relevance. Chores such as distributing laundry can be assigned to other staff members, rather than to nursing assistants. Also, employees must understand that although everyone has defined responsibilities, roles must become blurred at times (such as in transporting residents to and from a large activity such as a holiday celebration, or in interacting with residents on a routine basis). This can be facilitated by cross-training staff members. For example, nursing assistants can lead or assist with activities during "down time."

Facility Practices

Facilities may be organized differently to handle individuals with dementia. Some may have a special care unit, or units; others may not. If there are special care units, the criteria for admission and discharge or transfer must be clearly defined. In addition, family members need to be informed of these policies before admission. Facilities may have other special dementia programs as well, such as in-house day care, on-unit special programming, primary care nursing, and behavior teams. All staff should know the philosophy and criteria for these programs.

Team Building

A spirit of collaboration should be fostered. Opportunities for participation in care planning conferences and other decision-making activities need to be provided for various disciplines as well as all levels of staff. Staff should be recognized for their good work and disciplined when performance slacks off. To do their jobs supervisors and managers need ongoing training as well as administrative support. Professional growth should always be encouraged with support for staff to improve their knowledge and skills.

Training

Ongoing training should be provided for all disciplines and levels of facility staff. No matter how much training is provided, there can always be more. But because budgets are limited, strategic decisions must be made. Meeting minimal guidelines is often not enough. The issue of training nursing assistants is a good example. Although more professionalism has been accorded to nursing assistants by OBRA's mandate for their training, the 100 hours of required training is minimal. Basic curricular guidelines were set, but development and execution were left to the individual states; there is generally very little dementia-specific training. This basic minimum of formal training is to be supplemented by a specified minimum amount of required continuing education. This is a start, but often does not extend beyond the classroom. Frequently, there is little or no ongoing *informal* training. Studies have asserted that nursing assistants reported little or no opportunity to learn care skills from the nurses who are supervising them or from other members of the multidisciplinary staff. They also reported not feeling valued as members of the care planning team, in terms of not being asked for their opinions or input on resident care issues. For the majority of them, this contributes to their perception of being in a low-paying, dead-end job. Little attention has been paid to the development of a career ladder for nursing assistants.

If there is any common ingredient in the more successful dementia programs, it is the emphasis on staff training. Scope, content, and format of training are varied and require more research attention at this time.

Despite their education, licensure, and experience, many professional staff have not been taught much about dementia during their formal education and will require supplemental training on the job. Meanwhile, all staff members need to be provided with clear information regarding the facility's philosophy, programs, and procedures, as well as the skills necessary to implement them.

Staff Burnout: A Prevalent Problem

Burnout is a problem commonly ascribed to health care workers, many of whom work under stressful conditions. The stress ultimately results in health problems, diminished work efficacy, and staff turnover. Although nursing homes are chronic care facilities and function at a slower pace than acute care hospitals, where burnout is a prevalent concern, nursing home employees face many of the same risk factors for burnout.

Nursing home staff work with sick or terminal individuals, sometimes have life and death responsibilities, often feel helpless and defeated when patients' conditions worsen, work with residents who are stressed by their debilitation and are often nasty and resistant to care, and work within a highly regulated environment. In addition, they are out of the mainstream of health care. Further, they generally experience a minimum of training, receive relatively low monetary compensation, have a lack of prestige, and are given a paucity of resources with which to work and little emotional support. Moreover, a considerable proportion of their work is with demented patients, for whom providing care produces added stressors for the caregiver.

Working with demented residents involves frustrating resistances to care, verbal and physical lashing out, and residents' ultimate physical and mental deterioration despite competent and even heroic care efforts. There is little positive feedback from these residents, sometimes because of language dysfunctions. Ongoing training and skills improvement, team building, available information, emotional support, permanent and balanced assignments, personal health promotion programs, and

TABLE 3.1 Factors Associated With Burnout Prevention/Reduction

Administrative support
Information availability
Training/skills development
Positive reinforcement
Supervisory leadership
Team building
Encouragement of innovation
Permanent, balanced assignments for nursing assistants
Pleasant physical environments
Families incorporated into the care team

encouragement of staff to be flexible and innovative are important components of burnout prevention and stress reduction (Table 3.1).

Dementia and Health Care Reform: Future Directions

There is a demographic imperative to plan for the aging of the elderly population, who experience a range of associated frailties and disabilities, among which dementia is prevalent. Because of its pervasiveness, dementia is finally being recognized as an important social, health, and economic issue of the times. Although there have been multiple attempts at the development of funding streams for community services and some progress has been made, the widespread availability of appropriate, competent, and adequately funded services is still more a dream than a reality. The availability of expanded community services may, in fact, forestall nursing home placement and thus impact the type of institutional services needed.

The development of a systematic approach to care for demented nursing home residents is as yet in its infancy as well. Efforts are underway to begin to examine the concepts and components of specialized dementia care and to begin to measure their outcomes. Researchers and practitioners alike are searching for answers. Policymakers are awaiting better data as well. The following chapters will present information about a variety of directions and approaches that have been developed.

Suggested Reading

Aronson, M. K. (1993). Reducing stress in caregivers of dementia patients. In J. E. Jackson, R. Katzman, & P. J. Lessin (Eds.), *Alzheimer's disease: Long term care* (pp. 81-95). San Diego, CA: San Diego State University Press.

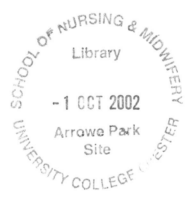

4

Approaches to Special Programming

Ronnie Grower
Cynthia Wallace
Gail Weinstein
Karen Lazar
Susan Leventer
Theresa Martico-Greenfield

The course of dementia is variable. There is an ebb and flow of behavioral symptoms. Pragmatically, this translates into a need for innovative and flexible programs. Specialized programs for individuals with dementia consider the needs and abilities of each individual. The structure of these programs creates the opportunity for stimulation and participation in a

AUTHORS' NOTE: Materials incorporated are also based on work by Polly V. DiCesare and Lucy Viti, Presbyterian Home for Central New York, New Hartford, NY; Vivian Dillon, Christine Horton, and Judith M. Scott, Morningside House, Bronx, NY; Michael N. Mulvihill, Jewish Home and Hospital for the Aged, New York, NY; and Taher Zandi, Alzheimer's Disease Assistance Center, Plattsburgh, NY.

TABLE 4.1 Elements of Dementia Programming

Philosophy and goals

Criteria for participants

Structure and consistency

Ongoing assessment

Adapted environment

Multidisciplinary team approach

Staff education/training/support

Modified activities/enriched program

Family involvement/support

Ongoing evaluation and feedback

supportive environment, where changes in the needs of participants can be identified and addressed.

This chapter will discuss examples of special programs designed to accommodate dementia patients. The programs presented were supported by the New York State Dementia Initiative. Several of the models have common elements (see Table 4.1). Although these programs have common elements, they differ in structure. They range from dedicated special units (Morningside and Presbyterian Houses), to centralized activities (the SHARE program), to a combination of the two (Jewish Home for Aged). The Kirkhaven Project is designed to enhance communication skills and can be used in any facility or setting. The last example is an attempt to ease the transition of patients from the community into nursing homes. Each of the models had an evaluation component (Table 4.2).

The tables in this chapter summarize the overall principles of these programs, including the basic components of programming, recommended activities and their goals, and variables

TABLE 4.2 Variables That May Be Used for Program Evaluation

Qualitative

Staff reactions

Family reactions

Quantitative

Level of resident participation in specified special program

Use of physical and chemical restraints

Added/diminished costs

Level of staff turnover

Measures of resident function

that can be used to evaluate programs. These concepts can be applied to any facility, whether or not a special dementia unit exists; in fact, they could usefully be incorporated into the fabric of all nursing homes.

Special Care Units

Morningside House Nursing Home

An Alzheimer's special care unit was created at Morningside House in the Bronx, New York, in 1977. This pioneering effort was designed to provide a therapeutic and secure environment for residents with moderately severe dementia with minimal use of psychotropic drugs and physical restraints. The salient features of this unit include modifications in the environment, organization of the staff into a multidisciplinary team, adaptation of activities to meet the needs of the patients, and an emphasis on ongoing staff training.

Environmental Adaptations

The environment in this Alzheimer's unit has carefully structured safe spaces that minimize disturbing stimuli and allow patients an opportunity for greater self-direction. Fluorescent lighting has been eliminated. Floors are carpeted, and a carpet panel placed along the corridor walls curtails the noise level.

Bothersome behaviors are channeled into more socially acceptable activities. For example, on the carpeted wall panel there are interesting shapes of Velcro-backed material that residents can move around at will, thus redirecting their perseverative actions. Similarly the tendency to rummage through the belongings of others has been transformed by creating a specially designed rummage area. Items in the rummage area include old clothing, hats, gloves, costume jewelry, photographs, kitchen utensils, and hobby equipment in drawers and cabinets that the residents are free to open, close, empty, and fill at any time.

The Team Approach

A unified team of staff from all levels and disciplines plays an important role in the lives of residents. The team concept promotes a high level of communication and interrelatedness. A staff organized in this way readily lends itself to developing a consistent and consolidated approach to patient care. Management of problem behaviors and deciphering residents' nonverbal cues or fragmented messages become a team challenge rather than an individual's burden. When verbal and nonverbal communications are understood by a caring staff, feelings of mutual trust and a sense of security grow.

Modified Activities

Program activities were modified and adapted to be sensitive to the cognitive, physical, and sensory deficits of the resi-

TABLE 4.3 Goals of Activities

Structure time

Keep patient physically active

Encourage mental stimulation

Provide setting for fun

Promote socialization

Facilitate opportunities for achievement

Improve self-esteem

Transform disease symptoms into purposeful activity

Enhance/reinforce skills

Maintain connections with others

Improve quality of life

---

dents. Goals of activities are summarized in Table 4.3. Adaptations include repetition and simplification of directions, multisensory stimulus presentation (including verbal and visual cuing), and task segmentation (i.e., dividing the activity into manageable single steps).

Functional ability is assessed on an ongoing basis in order to ensure that patients are appropriately challenged by the activities with a minimum of frustration. Activities that are repetitive and familiar and that utilize well-learned skills have been found to be most comfortable. For example, laundry is a task that nearly every patient has done in his or her lifetime. A "wash day," involving hanging and folding laundry, has been incorporated. Another strategy has been engaging individuals who have in the past had leadership roles. Activities for them include assisting staff in leading a group activity, assisting another resident during a program, or helping staff to develop or prepare materials for an event.

Staff Development

Ongoing education for the staff is essential. An initial 10-week series of weekly lectures and workshops gives the staff the skills they need to deal with the cognitively impaired residents and also provides a necessary support mechanism. Experiential workshops and refresher courses are ongoing for all staff members, no matter what level of experience they have.

Program Evaluation

Evaluation is another integral part of this program and is used as a tool for program modification and quality assurance. Qualitative outcomes are measured through feedback from families and staff observations of residents' level of participation, including verbal and nonverbal responses, attention span, and behavioral changes during the program. Features of this program have been replicated in many subsequent efforts.

Presbyterian Home of Central New York

In 1987 an existing 42-bed skilled nursing unit was converted into a special needs unit serving patients who had a primary diagnosis of dementia and were in the early and middle stages of the disease. The goals of this program were to "maintain the quality of life and dignity" of the patients and to reduce the use of chemical and physical restraints. The features are somewhat similar to those described previously, that is, a well-trained, multidisciplinary staff; a safe, stimulating environment for the patients; inclusion of residents' families in the team approach; and an enriched activities program. This program included clinical research tools for participant selection and program evaluation.

Selection of Residents

Program participants are either residents of the facility or registrants in the adult day services program. All are screened with the Special Needs Assessment Profile, which was based on Reisberg's Cognitive Function Scale and addressed activities of daily living (ADL) skills, cognition, wandering, social interaction, and speech deficits. It was determined that this instrument enabled selection of appropriate patients for the program.

Environmental Adaptations

Physical modifications include creating "memory" corridors and using pastel colors and textured walls. Corridor landmarks were provided to assist patients with way finding. In addition, corridors and outdoor areas were reconstructed so that residents are able to wander safely both indoors and out.

Enriched Activities

Enriched activity programs are designed to enhance and reinforce skills, such as self-feeding and grooming. Others are geared to improve socialization, such as the "coffee klatch." Language groups and physical activities are also important components. Resident autonomy is a hallmark of this program; residents are encouraged to determine for themselves whether or not they wish to participate. A menu of dementia-relevant activities is contained in Table 4.4.

Staffing

The unit staff were assembled from existing personnel in the nursing home facility. Staff from all disciplines worked together as a multidisciplinary team to develop and implement assessment methods and techniques and other program components. The family was integrated into the team from the outset.

Program Evaluation

Indications of this model's success are a low staff turnover rate and a stable unit population with a high occupancy rate.

TABLE 4.4 Activities That Are Relevant for Residents With Dementia

ADL-based

>   Grooming groups
>   Food preparation
>   Snacks
>   Shopping

Physical activities

>   Exercise/body awareness
>   Dancing
>   Walking clubs
>   Swimming (for those who have done this routinely)

Musical activities

>   Listening
>   Rhythm band
>   Singing
>   Playing an instrument
>   Musical games (e.g., Name That Tune)

Cognitive stimulation

>   Reminiscence
>   Reality orientation
>   Sensory awareness

Pet therapy

>   Visits from pets
>   Caring for resident pets (cats, dogs, birds, fish)
>   Visits to zoo
>   Bird watching

Games

>   Physical (ring toss, simplified basketball, parachute)
>   Word (spelling bees)
>   Other (bingo, horse racing)

Expressive activities

>   Psychodrama
>   Communication groups
>   Conversation

TABLE 4.4 (Continued)

Arts/crafts

Simple one-step tasks (task segmentation)
Collages

Intergenerational

Visits to or from children
Shared activities

Work oriented

Laundry day
Sheltered workshop
Gardening

Religious activities

Services
Pastoral visits
Rituals

Entertainment

Film classics
Musicals
Parties
Holiday celebrations
Seasonal activities

Providing continuity with past

Reminiscence
Props
Photo albums
Memorabilia
Encouraging accustomed roles (e.g., leadership)
Family visits

Rummaging

Socialization

Coffee klatches

In-House Day Care:
The SHARE Model

It is clear that the needs of individuals with dementia cover a broad spectrum. Special care units are not usually geared to those with very mild or severe impairments. Development of in-house day care has emerged as a model for middle-stage residents. Residents are taken off the unit for the bulk of their day and are involved in a specially structured program.

SHARE—Specialized Help for Alzheimer's in a Residential Environment—is an in-house day care at Morningside House. It was developed to accommodate moderately demented individuals, who were neither mainstreamed like the mildly demented nor placed in on-unit programs for the severely demented. Thus, this program is part of a continuum of dementia services within the facility. The program runs on weekdays from 9:30 a.m. to 3:30 p.m. Fifty residents are escorted from their units to a centralized area. There are discrete structured activity periods for socialization, toileting, lunch, and snacks.

Goals

This program offers a combination of nursing, social work, therapeutic recreation, and dietary and rehabilitation services. The goals of this program are to encourage association, recall, and reminiscence; provide a vehicle for thought and communication; promote socialization and a sense of purpose and belonging; reinforce appropriate behavior; maximize and maintain ADL skills; and facilitate environmental awareness and reality orientation in the patients.

Staffing

There is a program coordinator who supervises both the daily operations and the clinical aspects of the program. Nursing aides provide direct patient care and assistance during activities. There are also adjunct staff in the program from the departments of social work, occupational therapy, physical therapy, recreational therapy, dietary, nursing, and volunteers.

Participants

Program participants generally have a moderate dementia, but are able to engage in the program to some degree, do not require consistent one-on-one interventions for aberrant behavior, and are able to be escorted off the unit.

Program Format

The program follows a structured format, including welcoming/orientation, therapeutic activities, and meal and refreshment breaks. Therapeutic activities include cognitive and sensory stimulation, exercise and movement programs, music and rhythm, and reminiscence. Socialization is encouraged at all times. At lunchtime appropriate eating skills are featured. Lunch is followed by an unstructured activity or game. In good weather a popular activity is a short walk and rest period in the garden.

Evaluation

An evaluation of the SHARE program was conducted (Grower & Frazier, 1990). Forty-eight nursing home residents with dementia were randomly assigned to the SHARE program and a control group. Residents in the control group lived and interacted with cognitively intact residents and could elect to participate in the facility's daily recreational programs.

As with the evaluations of Alzheimer's programs in general, quantitative measures indicated that regardless of participation, residents with dementia deteriorated in the areas of manageability, self-care, orientation, depression, irritability, and sociability. Yet, qualitatively, the benefits of the SHARE program were evidenced by the endorsements of participants, staff, and families. Staff and families alike reported that participation in the program encouraged recall, humor, familiarity, and affection. In addition, this model allowed unit staff to get needed respite when some of the more difficult residents were attending the SHARE program off the unit.

The in-house day care program did not involve major structural renovations, but rather an allocation of programming space. Although capital costs were minimal, it required a financial commitment to add two staff members to coordinate, implement, and manage the day-to-day operations of the program. A nursing assistant was assigned to the program from the existing staff complement, so this was not an added cost for the facility but would be a consideration for facilities developing new programs.

A comparable program was tried at the Menorah campus in Buffalo, New York, and is described in the chapter by David M. Dunkelman and Randi C. Dressel. Results were similarly encouraging.

Nursing Unit-Based (Decentralized) Services: Jewish Home and Hospital for Aged

Because facilities differ in architecture and in size, different approaches to programming may be needed. Although 50 participants were found to be a manageable size in the above example, a similar program would not be feasible in a facility twice as large. At the Jewish Home and Hospital for Aged, a large, multistory facility in New York City, centralization of services was found to become unwieldy as residents aged in place and became demented and frail. Thus, this facility examined the effects of providing decentralized (that is, nursing unit-based) services to nursing home patients with dementia. The expectation was that offering meals and recreation programs on each floor would create a more intimate and comfortable environment for residents with dementia. Goals were to reduce stress for these residents and therefore to decrease agitation, reduce use of psychotropic medications, slow the decline in mental functioning, increase resident participation in recreation, and improve activities of daily living.

Program Description

The interventions in this program included three meals daily and recreation programs conducted on the residents' unit. By providing meals on the same unit, residents with dementia did not have to walk long distances and use an elevator to get to meals and were able to dine in a more intimate, less distracting environment. Thus, patients became less disoriented by staying in the environment with which they were most familiar.

Daily recreation programs on the decentralized care units included music, exercise, grooming, bingo, and horse racing. The programs took place in the day/dining room, thereby creating a less intimidating environment than the auditorium where activities normally occurred. Residents could come in and out of the program at will and remain safe in their familiar surroundings.

Evaluation

During the 2-year study period (1988-1990) four assessments were completed at 6-month intervals to detect if there were any changes in cognitive functioning, ADL status, and behavior as a result of the interventions. Four evaluation tools were used: the Mini-Mental State Exam, the Alzheimer's Disease Assessment Scale—both of which measure cognitive functioning; Barthel's Index, which measures activities of daily living; and the Nurses' Observation Scale for In-Patient Evaluation, which evaluates behavior.

Results from each of the four assessments showed little change in residents with dementia on both the demonstration and control floors. In addition, patterns of drug use in the control groups paralleled patterns of drug use in the intervention groups. Although not measurable by any of the research instruments utilized, anecdotal examples indicate that the experimental programs improved the quality of life of the residents.

Strategies for Maximizing Communication: The Kirkhaven Communication Project

The Kirkhaven Communication Project was a time-limited program that can be incorporated in any setting. It emphasized building up communication skills in patients to diminish isolation.

Program Description

An interaction model and assisted communication were used to produce improved performance (Leventer, 1992, p. 1). Communication groups were formed based on high, medium, and low communication abilities; those who were unable to speak were excluded. The project was founded on the premise that communication disorders increase feelings of isolation, exacerbate staff frustration, and deprive the individual with dementia of the benefits of interactions with team members, family, and volunteers.

The programs were based on the value of inclusion, the importance of which cannot be overemphasized. Whether on a one-to-one basis with the individual's primary (staff) caregiver or in the ongoing interactions in a group setting, the individual with dementia was afforded the opportunity to experience being part of a community. Participation was acknowledged and praised.

Groups consisted of five residents and five staff or family members and were time limited, meeting a total of 8 to 10 times. The primary goal of this labor-intensive program was "enhanced self-esteem for residents, and the acquisition of a core of communication skills for staff or family." Learning was not a goal for the residents.

Communication Strategies

The communication strategies used in the Kirkhaven project were specific:

1. Use of nonverbal cues and names to secure and maintain attention;
2. Use of FM amplifiers for selected residents who might benefit;
3. Focusing of conversations through the use of concrete objects;
4. Direct sentences, easy pace, repetition, and expansion of resident comments; and
5. "Conversation bridges" to change topics.

Residents' responses were measured in terms of 10 areas of performance including attention, comprehension, replies, initiation of conversation, and frequency of speech. Use of these five strategies resulted in major improvement in the residents' group communication skills. The percentage of residents who spoke more than three times in 30 minutes of group involvement increased from 31% to 98%. All 10 areas of response improved significantly.

Addressing Hearing Loss

Confounding the communication loss as dementia progresses is the loss of hearing associated with aging. All communication strategies must, therefore, take into account the complexity of hearing loss combined with neurological language impairment in dementia. Facing the patient at eye level, speaking rather than shouting, eliminating background noise, and reducing gestures that interfere with the patient's focus are effective communication strategies.

Social Day Care Program
as a Transition to Nursing Home Admission

Another issue that was addressed in the Dementia Initiative projects was easing the transition from home to nursing home by using a social day care program whereby the amount of time spent at the facility is increased gradually.

Program Description

This model uses a social day care program as the means to ease the transition from home to nursing home. One of the project's aims was to create a "triangle of care" involving the patients, their families, and the nursing home staff. This was found to lead to better adjustment of the residents.

Evaluation

Residents were evaluated using the Cambridge Examination for Mental Disorders of the Elderly, Reisberg's Brief Cognitive Rating and Functional Assessment Scales, and Zandi's Social Observed Behavior Scale. Residents who participated in a social day care program showed remarkably better social abilities and adjusted better to the nursing home placement than those residents who did not participate in this program and went directly into the nursing home. It must be noted that there is a possible sampling bias in that those who chose not to participate in the social day program served as a control group.

Conclusion

The success of specialized programming for dementia patients depends on a highly structured environment, a nonthreatening atmosphere of acceptance and understanding, maximum communication, and the delivery of services by well-trained, motivated, and caring staff. Until Alzheimer's disease is eradicated, nursing care facilities must provide a continuum of services and support, as well as appropriate programming and dedication to increased knowledge and awareness—all of which are part of the fabric of quality of life and quality of care.

References

Grower, R., & Frazier, C. (1990, April). *Applying a community based day care program to a nursing home setting.* Paper presented at the Northeastern Gerontological Society Conference, New Haven, CT.

Leventer, S. (1992, January). *Communication in dementia: strategies for success: A demonstration project.* Paper presented at the Jewish Guild for the Blind Health Facilities Corporation Workshop, Yonkers, NY.

Suggested Readings

Aronson, M. (1982). Alzheimer's disease: An overview. *Generations, 7,* 6-7.

Coons, D., & Weaverdyck, S. W. (1986). Wesley Hall: A residential unit for persons with Alzheimer's disease and related disorders. A therapeutic intervention for the person with dementia [Special issue]. *Physical & Occupational Therapy in Geriatrics, 4*(3), 29-53.

Katz, M. M. (1976). Behavioral change in the chronicity pattern of dementia in the institutional geriatric resident. *Journal of the American Geriatrics Society, 24,* 522-528.

Lubinski, R. (Ed.). (1991). *Dementia and communication.* Hamilton, Ontario: B. C. Decker.

Reisberg, B. (1983). *Alzheimer's disease: The standard reference.* New York: Free Press.

5

The Nursing Home Environment and Dementia Care

David M. Dunkelman
Randi C. Dressel

The central paradox of Alzheimer's is that although it is a brain disease, it manifests itself socially in behavior. For its victims, it twists and misshapes the world and all its related parts. One way to discuss the nursing home care implications of Alzheimer's is to tease apart the interrelated variables of the physical environment, the caregiving program, and the costs involved.

For too long the relationship between nursing home building and program has not been studied and their interdependency has been ignored. Instead, consultants who know nothing about the resident, the worker, the family, or their day together have been requested to "design." The environment created is generally regarded as state of the art, and the design often leaves the users with a less than optimal structure they must work around for many years. This chapter will challenge the reader to examine the elements of an appropriate physical environment for dementia care.

John Hull's book *Touching the Rock* describes the pheno-menological experience of blindness, an experience that may serve as a paradigm for dementia. Hull describes how not only the function of the outer eye but also that of the "inner eye" gradually vanishes with blindness. The damage to the visual apparatus of the eye affects the visual area of the brain, which ultimately results in the loss of all visual concepts, thinking, and identity. In such cases neurologists speak of cortical blindness, of central or ideational blindness, and of not being able even to reconstruct the memory of one's own face. Hull also describes heightened phantasmal visual images that may occur as the person descends into blindness—terrifying hallucinations akin to the phantom limbs amputees feel and the phantasmal voices that accompany deafness.

One idea that can be extracted from this book is the exist-ence of a very direct connection between the mind and body. In essence, the mind is a dedicated processor that makes the body's actions and experiences real. This reverses Woody Allen's adage that the brain is his second favorite organ. In the context of this discussion, this is particularly frightening when one thinks of Alzheimer's disease. Alzheimer's destroys the brain and appears to do so in a seemingly random manner. Imagine the brain as a bunch of ripe grapes. Words and ideas are contained within the grapes. As each sack of information loses integrity, the sack walls retain less, eventually drying out and withering, able to hold nothing.

Hull's book leads to a second idea, that the brain may be capable of dimensions of thought and experience that humans cannot contemplate. Given the malfunction and mistransmis-sion in the mind of the Alzheimer's patient, who knows the fabric, the texture, and the tenor of the patient's experiences? An integral part of the progression of Alzheimer's disease may be the brain's search for proper connections to the body. This phenomenon may be responsible for the cognitive fantasies, stimulus misinterpretations, and other unpredictable behaviors characteristic of demented individuals. This suggests that the physical environment of a health care facility for the elderly should support as wide a range of behaviors as possible. Yet the design of most nursing homes does not accomplish this. To date, available solutions have been somewhat limited for a number of reasons.

First, design is difficult because the parameters of dementia itself are vague. There is limited instrumentation, let alone outcome measures. The disease gets progressively worse, and behaviors are intermittent and somewhat unpredictable. Thus, in actuality, little data have been developed on which new design approaches can be built.

Second, there is confusion as to for whom the facility is being designed. Many of the nursing home issues involving Alzheimer's patients—for example, locked and segregated units, shared rooms, and tracking technologies—revolve around efficiency, convenience, and safety for the patients, staff, other residents, and administration. All of these parties should be considered part of the client cluster group. It would be fruitful to analyze and meet the specific needs of each group, rather than to do so covertly under the guise of addressing resident needs.

A third problem involves the amount of stimulation to be experienced by the patients. Because architecture tends to focus around visual issues, it frequently fails to properly address the other senses. The cognitively impaired individual is more susceptible to external stimuli and distractions than his or her nondemented counterpart. Thus, auditory, tactile, and olfactory cues may have significant impact on behavior. This suggests that many of the frequently cited Alzheimer's design issues such as color, furniture style, and electronic monitoring devices may miss the point.

Many of the stimuli that are problematic to an individual with dementia are masked to the nondemented person. Unable to filter out the voice of a paging system, the motion of a medication cart, or the general bustle of the highly modern nursing unit, the dementia patient's attention continually shifts, interrupting fragile trains of thought and causing frustration—a frustration not easily recognized by others who have not experienced the problem.

Human Costs

A different way of looking at the nursing home care environment may be based on productivity and cost—not financial cost, but human cost to the aide or the resident for each task. Alzheimer's disease creates an internal unpredictability, often amplified by environmental unpredictability. Certain experiences tend to elicit stressful responses from the resident. Each of these responses is costly in terms of emotional discomfort and heightened care needs. A nursing assistant knows that having to walk distances with an agitated Alzheimer's patient has a high cost. She also knows that random stimulation by noise and/or physical bustle also has high costs. For the under-trained aide, the cost of living moment-to-moment with the unpredictability of the behaviors frequently forces him or her to retreat—to cut off feelings or emotional investment. Thus, there is a compounding or deepening of costs for both resident and caregiver.

To the nursing assistant, the demented individual's response to overperceived stimuli may appear to be dangerous. The intuitive intervention is to inhibit this behavior, either with physical or chemical restraints. As a result, the patient is suddenly faced with a whole new set of incomprehensible stimuli: side effects from the medication and/or devices that rob control over body movements. The ensuing frustration may cause more frightened and frightening behavior, which in turn may result in the use of even more restraints. The cycle continues. The loss of movement resulting from restraints produces other symptoms, such as the reduction of muscle tone, skin integrity, appetite, peristalsis, bone density, and balance. Thus many of today's additional costs are iatrogenic. Ultimately, there is a downward spiral that seems inevitable and unrelenting. The caregivers are discouraged by the hopelessness of the situation. This therapeutic nihilism disengages the last supporters and advocates from the patient.

An additional cost of the patient's increased agitation is the family's growing struggle with guilt, anger, and terror from the accompanying downward spiral of their loved one and their desperate search for meaning. They sense that there is an underlying equation that, if rediscovered, would explain their relative's behaviors. It is almost as if they had merely lost the legend and symbols to a map.

Architecture Reconsidered

A logical response to these dementia care problems would be to think on a smaller scale and to build small-scale, quiet and less stimulating environments, designed for stimulation from the natural elements (sun, moon, rain, etc.) and for carefully controlled, individualized routines. The ideal physical environment would be the antithesis of the typical nursing home, whose medicalized routines and reimbursement systems call out for quickened rhythms and bursts of activities and for larger scale batch processing rather than individualization. The behaviors elicited in this latter environment may enormously exaggerate the symptoms and ultimately increase the cost of the disease.

The proper role of architecture should be considered in light of the very unique problems presented by this disease. In a sense, architecture has been viewed backwards. The secret to design for the Alzheimer's victim is not to create an environment but to create a human experience.

In-House Day Care: A Program Example

An example of an attempt to create a human experience for nursing home residents with Alzheimer's disease was the development of an in-house Alzheimer's (social) day care program at the Rosa Coplon Home in Buffalo, New York. The program resulted from a grant proposal to identify and explore effective management and environmental techniques for working with people with mental impairments.

Once it was determined that an in-house day care would be developed, a series of assessments was done. Methods of classification and determining appropriate candidates for the program were evaluated. Measurement instruments were identified and used, which included the Folstein Mini-Mental Status Examination and the Haycox Dementia Behavior Scale. A "tool kit" was developed with a full complement of instruments that fit with the program's notions of cognitive functioning. Some instruments were used directly with the patients; others involved caregivers. Clients with little or no impairments received a distinct set of questions from those with mild to moderate impairments. As a result of these assessments, it was determined that the residents in need of dementia programs resided throughout the facility. Thus, it was decided that a central location for programming would be best.

The activity room was chosen as the location for the day care program and 20 residents were selected to participate. The day care program ran from 10:00 a.m. to 3:00 p.m., Monday through Friday. A program assistant scheduled the day's activities, including social programs, memory groups, cognitive skills, and exercises. The program assistant was joined each day by a nursing assistant, who was assigned from another unit in the facility. A nurse assisted for one hour during mealtime, and activities and other staff assisted with programming throughout the day. All medications were brought to the day care location for dispensing.

The program assistant was responsible for progress notes on a quarterly basis, for the leisure activity program requirements, for completing behavior and activities for daily living (ADL) tracking forms for nursing, and for attending all unit-based care planning meetings. A care plan card was maintained for each individual in the program.

Program Impact

The day care program made an impact on the residents, the staff, and the institution itself. The residents received more specialized treatment, were observed to be less restless and more responsive in day care, and were found to interact with others more spontaneously. In addition, resident competencies were discovered, that is, people began feeding themselves, communicating, and recapturing memory, which was not evident on the units.

The nursing units became quieter and more manageable. Because many of the residents who wandered and called out were now off the unit during the day, the unit became a less demanding environment that increased staff morale and efficiency. Moreover, the Alzheimer's day care staff knew the clients' individual patterns better and were trained to meet these individualized needs. These successes provided examples for other facility staff.

In addition to training those aides specifically working in the day care itself, this program effectively trained the entire facility's staff. By giving the day care staff special training, the remaining staff on the units felt left out. Unit staff rotated through day care and, therefore, each aide slowly learned skills and concepts that were then carried back to the units. After an initial adjustment period, the families liked the day care—they felt that their loved ones were getting special attention and that the environment was more quiet and less disruptive and upsetting to them.

Implications for Nursing Home Practice

Rearrangement of space. For a variety of reasons the traditional building is no longer adequate to provide appropriate, integrated care for the Alzheimer's patient. By taking residents with dementia to a central day care program, an appropriate social space was created for them. Additionally, refurbishing the activities room was much less expensive than refurbishing the units. The in-house day care model more appropriately addresses the special needs of this population and overcomes a number of limitations of the traditional buildings.

Meeting the needs of a changing population. The traditional nursing home building was designed for a more ambulatory, cognitively intact, self-caring population. Generally, the floors centered around a residential-bedroom concept where people would go downstairs for programming. With the aging in place of the population, frail nonambulatory people could no longer leave their units for activities. This created a dilemma. There was insufficient social space on the units, and there were too many residents for individualized programming. Ironically, the downstairs common spaces were underutilized.

Balancing of case loads. Taking certain residents off the unit reduced patient density and made the nursing floor unit more manageable. Ambulatory patients with mild to moderate dementia require extensive staff effort that, if not paced appropriately, can be a precipitant of staff burnout.

Reversal of therapeutic nihilism. Because of ingrained attitudes, there is a therapeutic nihilism at work—a sense that nothing can be done and that expended energy is useless. By placing the patient and caregiver in a special environment, with special training to overcome this negativism, progress has been perceived and measured, leading to a sense of accomplishment.

Developing new staff behaviors. Because the day care program is on a small scale, has a small staff, and is in a new place, an entirely new set of tasks and routines have been established without redoing old routines. In addition, only a few people had to be trained initially. By developing a day care program of excellence, rotating other staff through the program can get them to learn what can be done. New behaviors and attitudes can be stimulated and reinforced.

Wider inclusion of residents in programs. In traditional
nursing homes, designing a program on a bed or unit base
would require constantly moving residents on and off the floor
as their functioning changes. This is disruptive to residents,
families, and staff. The unit-based problem can be eliminated
by an in-house social day care program that does not need to
move patients from their sleeping rooms. Thus, the program
can include individuals from the entire facility, who can continue their old sleeping and nursing arrangements while participating.

Conclusion

In-house day care is an expedient intervention given limited
facilities and financial resources for change. Other residential
approaches have been tried, including a host of special care
units. To date, the efficacy of special units has not been demonstrated. Further research is sorely needed. Program development must take into account not only space and cost issues but
the delicate interrelationships and overlaps between these variables and the fragile individual for whom the services are
intended.

Suggested Readings

Haycox, J. A. (1984). A simple, reliable clinical behavioral scale for assessing
    demented patients. *Journal of Clinical Psychiatry, 45*(1), 23-24.
Hull, J. M. (1990). *Touching the rock: An experience of blindness.* New York:
    Pantheon.

6

Families as an Integral Part of Dementia Care

Patricia Gaston

Alzheimer's disease is a progressive illness with a course that may span many years. During this time both the afflicted individuals and their families go through a series of transitions and role changes. Family members often make great sacrifices to provide "quality of environment" for their loved one.

Most individuals with Alzheimer's disease and other dementias are cared for at home by their families for much of the course of their illness. However, as time goes on the patient's care needs change in nature and intensity; they can do less and less and have an increasingly difficult time communicating their needs. Caregiving strategies that once may have worked are no longer useful. For many families, the escalating and unrelenting physical and psychological demands of caregiving reach a point when the dreaded realization that "it's time" must be confronted.

The Placement Decision

Families generally seek nursing home placement as a last resort, either when they are overwhelmed by the patient's care needs, the caregiver's health is severely compromised, or home care without any financial assistance is no longer feasible. Deciding on placement for a loved one with dementia often represents an emotionally difficult choice. In the placement process, family members experience a range of often conflicting and painful feelings. Anger, guilt, relief, abandonment, and a sense of personal defeat or loss of control are perhaps the most common. These psychologically distressing feelings often persist during and after placement.

A decision to place a family member in an institution does not necessarily reduce caregiver burden. Family members are often forced to make this difficult decision when they are physically, emotionally, and financially exhausted (Gwyther, 1988). A flood of images, both real and imagined, may begin to cloud their judgment as they prepare for placement. Questions abound. How will they take care of my husband? Will they know what to do when my mother becomes agitated? How can I ever let go? The nursing home can be a source of support. Imagined, often horrifying, images can be replaced by clear, realistic ones. The nursing home can become an extension of home rather than a feared prison or sterile institution.

For many families readiness and acceptance may never be truly realized. The primary caregivers (often elderly spouses, siblings, or adult children—mostly daughters) need emotional support and psychological guidance during the placement process. They may seek this support from many sources, including family, friends, nursing home staff, their physician, and their local Alzheimer's Association chapter.

Many nursing homes have been responding to the unique and special care needs of dementia patients and their families. Special care units (SCUs) have grown in popularity, with a recent estimate that these units are operating in approximately 10% of nursing homes. In addition, institutions that have no discrete dementia units have adapted many of their general policies and procedures to better accommodate the needs of these patients and their families. One of the major adaptations is a greater emphasis on recognizing and addressing the emotional needs of families. A therapeutic plan is developed for both patient and family. This chapter will address issues that come up when families deal with nursing home care and therapeutic management of the dementia patient.

OBRA and the Admissions Process

OBRA legislation addressed "requirements for and assuring quality of care in skilled nursing facilities." Although the reforms and subsequent requirements did not address the needs of the demented or any other specific groups of residents, the reforms with regard to admissions, assessments, and care planning are certainly applicable.

OBRA requires that there be a preadmission screening to assure that mentally ill and mentally retarded individuals receive active treatment for their problems, rather than placement in a nursing home. Alzheimer's disease and other forms of dementing illness have been recognized as exceptions for this admission exclusion. However, the necessity for this screening should encourage persons with dementia symptoms to receive a diagnostic workup to assure that no reversible condition exists.

A comprehensive and reproducible assessment must be done on admission; this assessment must be repeated yearly. It must also be done when and if there are any significant changes in the patient's functioning or health status. A briefer quarterly review is required as well. The expanded assessment process was designed to positively impact care planning and implementation for all residents. Systematic care planning with the participation of residents, where feasible, and their family members or designated representatives, is required, with the goal of improving quality of care and quality of life.

Family Involvement
in the Admissions Process

Families appear at the doorsteps of nursing homes in extremely vulnerable and compromised emotional states. They are frightened and apprehensive about what will happen to their loved one. They are also, in fact, frightened about what will happen to them once they relinquish their full-time caregiving role that, for many, was all consuming. The nursing home staff must be acutely sensitive to the fragility of the family members and actively engage them in the admissions process without overburdening them. How can this delicate balance be achieved?

The staff must realize that first impressions are important. What families feel, sense, see, smell, and hear determine their opinions of how a nursing home cares for its residents. Staff interactions with residents, other staff, and families are closely observed. Families listen for language and communication styles and tune into body language and nonverbal cues as well. These variables may contribute toward (or hinder) a successful outcome and must be considered.

The Preadmission Phase

The preadmission phase generally includes the initial visit or tour of the facility (usually without the patient), the application process, and then (in many facilities) an interview with the patient and primary caregiver/family member(s). In addition to the family member(s), home attendants may be called on for specific information related to the patient's functioning. Given time constraints and financial pressures, many institutions have significantly curtailed this preadmission phase. However, it is important to note that this process allows families sufficient opportunities to get acquainted with the staff as well as to get a feel for the facility. The family will be asked to provide information about the patient: his or her background, interests, preferences, and premorbid personality style and habits. Staff may also request a medical/neurological disease-specific profile (including age of onset, diagnostic workup, and findings); description of the progression, abilities, and limitations related to activities of daily living (ADL); and information about appetite, sleep patterns, medications, and behaviors including agitation and other symptoms specific to dementing illness.

Families may also be asked about their successful and unsuccessful caregiving strategies and behavioral interventions, especially during episodes of agitation. The information from the family simultaneously provides important and necessary information for the hands-on nursing staff and a shared feeling of concern for the patient. This relationship and cooperative partnership help to create and facilitate a familiar and comfortable therapeutic environment. Most important, it acknowledges the caregiver's continued role as "expert" and reminds them that their opinions count. The link between patient and family need not be severed as a result of placement. The caregiver role is not totally relinquished, but rather shared. The physical demands of caregiving are passed onto the new caregivers—the facility staff.

Admission Day

Admission day has been described by many family caregivers as "the worst day of their lives." Patients often sense an ensuing change and can become agitated and upset, although they may have forgotten their preadmission visit. Families tend to set their internal barometers on how their loved ones ease into this change. Given the unpredictability that accompanies Alzheimer's disease, an aura of uncertainty prevails.

An integral part of easing the transition for the family and patient is knowing that the nursing home staff is ready for their relative and possesses some basic information. The patient is no longer a stranger; he or she is respectfully welcomed and immediately becomes engaged. Families should be encouraged to spend as much time as possible during the initial transition. Moving in can be slow and gradual. Adjustment is a process that takes time and cannot be rushed. Some dementia units have extended their admissions process to include a gradual transitions from day care. The patient and family slowly ease their way in: initially for 4 hours a day, then 8 hours, then overnight. This deliberate attempt to gradually admit a dementia patient addresses the patient's potentially heightened suspiciousness and accompanying paranoia with new situations.

Admission day is itself a process. The physical act of escorting an Alzheimer's disease patient to the nursing home may present problems. Agitation, fear of the unknown, and physical resistance may be encountered. Faced with these practical problems and the emotional drain, families are asked to collect and pack their loved one's life in a suitcase. To compound the problems, families are often notified of an opening in a nursing home 24 hours prior to admission.

A nursing home admission for a person with dementia is labor intensive, time-consuming, and emotionally draining. A significant amount of time during the first day is spent with the social worker and family reviewing institutional policies and procedures and filling out forms. Family members often feel so emotionally and physically depleted that they feel ill the next day. Often they require several days to recover psychologically from their traumatic first day's experience. Acclimation to the new environment may better occur over several days or even weeks, for example, meeting with unit staff and participating in care planning.

Thus, the concept of admission needs to be reconsidered. Although some things can best be accomplished during the preadmission phase, many of the important patient-related tasks must be left for the actual moving in. For example, setting up the patient's room with familiar memorabilia can be accomplished during the first week. As the patient is beginning to settle in and becomes more comfortable, he or she can assist with organizing and setting up the room. Active participation becomes a meaningful and purposeful task instead of another burden that families have to endure. Generally, over time the patient and his or her belongings will be assimilated into the new surroundings; this will help provide a more personalized and homelike atmosphere.

Easing the Transition: Family and Staff Interaction

As the patient and family become more familiar with the nursing home's routine, staff, and approach to care and management, the initial transitional anxiety begins to fade. The treatment team (consisting of the physician, nurse, nursing assistants, dietitian, activities therapist, and social worker), are actively working toward building trusting, caring relationships with families. Fostering these positive relationships takes time and hard work. Part of this therapeutic relationship includes keeping the lines of communication open. Exchange of information and ideas lead to mutually agreed on techniques, plans, and goals. Staff and family work as a team to effect a successful adjustment and enrich the care and quality of life for the resident with dementia. The resident, above all, is comforted and supported by a consistent approach.

Although some families find sufficient relief merely in not having 24-hour responsibilities for their demented relative, some do not. They have continuing concerns about the quality and adequacy of ongoing institutional care and their new role. Just as the care needs of the dementia patient continue after institutionalization, so, too, do the needs of the families. For many caregivers the period following nursing home placement may be as stressful as the years of caregiving, or even more so. Visiting may be difficult and burdensome, and interacting with staff may create problems. In addition, the nursing home environment can be quite disturbing for family members to observe. Commonly, on admission, families tend to feel that the other patients are "much sicker" than their relative, no matter what his or her actual condition (Kahan, 1984).

Support Groups for Families

Support groups have emerged as the most common vehicle for emotional support. Key components of a family support group include information, education, and problem solving, all shared and processed in a mutually supportive and nonjudgmental atmosphere. Many institutions have incorporated family support groups into their program.

In nursing homes, family support groups are usually led by a social worker. The spirit of a support group is community; an accepting place/atmosphere where feelings, even forbidden wishes (such as wishing the patient dead) can be openly expressed and supported. Friendships can be fostered. Complaints or concerns can be channeled in hopes of creating a more accepting and positive response from direct care staff. Meeting each other's expectations realistically and supportively is essential. Educating and helping families effectively negotiate with nursing home staff is another therapeutic goal for a support group.

Roles of Families After Placement

What do families do after placement? Once the patient has adjusted to the new surroundings, what next? Families repeatedly ask themselves, "How do I fit in now? What is my new role?" The nursing home can help family members identify their own needs and define their changed roles.

The nursing home and its staff must provide an environment in which families feel welcome and part of life in the facility. Many homes have developed pamphlets or other guides to aid families during the adjustment period and beyond. Others have adapted their procedures and practices. For example, maintaining unrestricted visiting hours or open visitation is an important strategy. In this way families do not feel restricted by prescribed visiting hours. Essentially, they are not considered visitors, but rather part of the fabric of the units on which their loved ones reside.

Visiting a loved one with dementia is frequently a lonely experience for many family members. The staff can be helpful in providing guidance. Families should be advised to consider the unit's routine and schedule of activities. Coordinated visits with other patients' families may help to minimize isolation and loneliness. Some families may enjoy visiting during an activities program and participating with their loved ones. Performing short, purposeful tasks (for example, grooming or walking) during visits can also help reduce the stressfulness of the visit, given the dementia patients' short attention spans and other cognitive deficits.

Families often want to offer their services and ask staff what they can do to work collaboratively toward a common goal. An important opportunity for such collaboration is in assisting with activities programs. Families can also supplement the activity program by lending their special talents to the group. Programs facilitated by families can be an enriching experience for everyone, as can unexpected environmental amenities such as pictures or furnishings or flowers, for example.

There are instances where family members cannot be actively involved on a day-to-day basis; however, attendance of family support groups and patient care conferences can assist these families by giving them a purposeful role. What is most important is the message that is communicated: Families are an integral member of the caring team. They are invited to become members of a new, extended family. Promoting and fostering an ongoing staff-family team approach to patient care creates an environment of warmth and acceptance for the Alzheimer patient. The patient begins to feel that everyone—their loved ones and their new extended nursing home family—cares about them.

Emotional Support for Staff

Caregiving is a physically and emotionally exhausting job. Family caregivers and nursing home staff members share many of the same concerns and experiences. Some, however, are unique to each group. Institutions have become more sensitive to the emotional needs of their staff. Management has recognized the pitfalls and problems that are created when staff, particularly nursing staff, becomes overburdened.

Burnout is a commonly used term in the health care industry. Traditionally, long-term care settings have been most vulnerable. Nursing home staff members are particularly at risk for burnout. It is stressful to nurse terminally ill patients with whom long-standing interpersonal caregiving relationships have been established. Moreover, there is little, if any at all, positive feedback. The dementia team, by definition, cares for patients with difficult and often unpredictable behaviors, which may create or exacerbate the psychological needs of the caring individuals and require interventions for them as well. The patients are truly not served if the needs of the staff are ignored. (Edelson & Lyons, 1985).

Staff support is an ongoing process that requires continual effort and commitment. It does not end after an extensive training or in-service program. Teaching, modeling, and supervision are hallmarks of a successful therapeutic approach for staff. The team leader, whether a nursing care coordinator or social worker, creates a trusting, collaborative environment. An effective dementia team works collaboratively and supportively. Roles are often blurred and expanded. Flexibility (or "going with the flow") is built in and expected. Line staff, typically considered the lowest persons on the totem pole, are made to feel important and involved and are assured that their opinions count. Not surprisingly, this involvement parallels the family member's experience.

Support groups can facilitate an open dialogue between and among staff. These groups are not structured like group therapy but rather serve as an arena for discussion, ventilation, mutual support, and problem solving. Management must make a time investment so that groups must be scheduled regularly. Ongoing training should also be included. A case presentation, for example, can be utilized to highlight specific behavioral interventions that may or may not be effective. Establishing positive staff working relationships can be a natural outcome of such a group experience as well.

In addition, staff support must be provided individually. Praising someone's accomplishments, regardless of how seemingly minor, should be done by the supervisor and unit leader on a continuous basis. Direct reassurances and support for behavioral interventions that may have proven unsuccessful can still offer a staff member a feeling of acknowledgment and importance. Flexibility in scheduling unit responsibilities and patient care assignments can go a long way toward successful team building and goal attainment.

In summary, dealing with the resident who has dementia involves not only care of the afflicted individual but care of the caregivers as well. Dementing illness is a long malignant process that exacts a toll not only on the patient but on those on whom the patient depends for survival. Once the patient is placed, support must be provided not only for the family members but for the institutional caregivers as well.

References

Edelson, J. S., & Lyons, W. H. (1985). *Institutional care of the mentally impaired elderly.* New York: Van Nostrand Reinhold.

Gwyther, L. P. (1988). *Nursing home care Issues.* In M. K. Aronson (Ed.) & staff of the Alzheimer's Disease and Related Disorders Association, *Understanding Alzheimer's disease* (pp. 238-262). New York: Charles Scribner's Sons.

Kahan, J. S. (1984). *The effects of a group support approach in decreasing feelings of burden and depression in relatives of patients with Alzheimer's disease and other dementing illness.* Unpublished doctoral dissertation, U.S. International University, San Diego, CA.

Suggested Readings

Aronson, M. K. (Ed.), & Alzheimer's Disease and Related Disorders Association Staff. (1988). *Understanding Alzheimer's disease.* New York: Charles Scribner's Sons.

Blevins, E. L., Darrell, L. J., & Bonedrake, C. L. (1987). *The nursing home and you: Partners in caring for a relative with Alzheimer's disease.* Washington, DC: American Association of Home for the Aging.

Friends and Relatives of the Institutionalized Aged, Inc. (1992). *A family guide to effective participation in comprehensive care planning.* New York: Author.

Gwyther, L. (1985). *Care of Alzheimer's patients: A manual for nursing home staff.* Washington, DC: American Health Care Association & Alzheimer's Disease and Related Diseases Association.

New York City Department for the Aging Residential and Nursing Home Affairs Unit. (1988). *Initial contacts with families of dementia patients: A guide for residential health care facilities staff.* New York: Author.

Ronch, J. L. (1989). *Alzheimer's disease: A practical guide for those who help others.* New York: Continuum.

7

Strategies for Management of Behavioral Problems

Miriam K. Aronson

Dementia involves an interplay of cognitive, functional, and behavioral symptoms. Cognitive symptoms include declines in memory, judgment, orientation, language, abstract reasoning, and problem-solving abilities. These difficulties affect the ability to perform routine daily activities, such as bathing, dressing, grooming, toileting, and eating. The functional declines may cause frustration, which may produce behavioral problems, or may be compounded by other associated behavioral dysfunctions.

The care for most demented individuals is provided at home by families, who continue their caregiving for many years until they become overwhelmed. The patient's health and personal care needs grow as the disease progresses and the level of dysfunction increases. Placement of loved ones in a nursing home is usually a last resort. The functional and behavioral deterioration that precipitated placement continue after admission and must be dealt with by nursing home staff. This chapter will focus on the behavioral aspects of dementia and associated care needs.

Dementia-Associated Behaviors

Dementia-associated behaviors include agitation, wandering, sleep-wake disturbances, paranoia, hallucinations, verbal and physical aggression, sexual inappropriateness, apathy, catastrophic reactions, and general resistance to care. Depression is a frequent comorbidity. Some researchers have labeled these sequelae "disruptive behaviors" because this term reflects the interaction between the actual behavior and the emotions of the caregiver who is perceiving it as a problem (Jackson, Drugovich, Fretwell, Spector, Sternberg, & Rosenstein, 1989). Other researchers have described disruptive behaviors among the cognitively impaired as agitation. I will call them behavioral sequelae to use a more neutral term.

Behavioral sequelae are prevalent in individuals with dementia. About half of a cohort of community-residing patients with mild dementia had one behavioral symptom; the prevalence rose to 80% for those with severe illness. The pattern was similar for the group with two or more symptoms, with a range from 32% to 70% (Eisdorfer, Cohen, Paveza, Ashford, Luchins, et al. 1992). Two other studies found a comparable prevalence in patients with three or more symptoms, 20% (Teri, Larson, & Reifler, 1992) and 27% (Cohen, Eisdorfer, Gorelick, Paveza, Luchins, et al., 1993). Symptom patterns appear to be associated with severity of illness and also to subtypes of dementia, such as multi-infarct dementia.

Behavioral symptoms are almost ubiquitous in nursing homes. Reports of prevalence of behavioral disturbances in nursing home patients have ranged from 22.6% (Rovner, German, Broadhead, Morriss, Brant, et al., 1990) to 76% (Zimmer, Watson, & Treat, 1984). The variation in these figures is attributable to differences in study definitions and methodology. Accurate data are needed for planning and development of programs appropriate to this population.

Sundowning

Sundowning is a dementia-associated behavioral dysfunction whereby the level of confusion and associated agitation seems to increase markedly in the late afternoon or early evening. Sundowning is a clinical hallmark of the intraindividual variability of the dementia patient. It should be noted that results of functional assessments performed late in the afternoon may differ remarkably from those done earlier in the day.

Although sundowning probably has a biological substrate, its manifestations may be somewhat alterable by programmatic adjustments. Management of the sundowning phenomenon is especially difficult in the nursing home because it challenges current practices. Traditionally, staffing is less on the evening shift than the day shift and still less at night. An important feature of dementia-specific programming, therefore, is the modification of the number and type of staff available during the late afternoon and other times of increased need.

Although the major part of activities programming occurs during the day in most facilities, intensified late afternoon/early evening activities programming is required to rechannel agitated behaviors. For the physically active, pacing may be redirected into walking or dancing. For others, noisiness may be channeled into singing or a rhythm band. Because of increased restlessness, added staffing may be needed during dinner as well as modifications of the menu to include more finger foods for faster service. Those residents using psychotropic medications for target symptoms that seem to have a temporal pattern may require adjustments of dosage and time of administration so their peak effect coincides with the most severe symptoms.

Sleep-Wake Disturbance

Difficulties with orientation extend beyond the individual's inability to tell time. As the dementia progresses, changes may occur in the sleep-wake cycle. Patients may become restless at night and may experience insomnia. Depression, which often accompanies dementia, may cause sleep disturbances as well. Increasing the night staff would allow sleepless patients to roam safely under supervision, as well as to utilize available activities materials and wandering space on a 24-hour basis. Insomnia may also be selected as a target symptom for other behavioral and/or pharmacologic interventions.

Catastrophic Reactions

Individuals with dementia may overreact to, or become disproportionately upset by, stimuli or situations that do not warrant these behaviors. Catastrophic reactions are often unpredictable, although occasionally there are identifiable precipitants. These may include specific activities such as bathing, dressing, or grooming; being involved in new or strange situations; being asked to do something that is beyond their capabilities; being visited by a particular individual; or having to leave the unit or the building for an appointment.

Staff must be to trained to recognize that these behaviors are not intentional, but rather the effects of a failing brain, and must intervene appropriately. First, identification of precipitants can help to avoid or lessen the problem. For example, if bathing is a traumatic event, perhaps the presence of a favorite staff member or a loved one could ease the problem. If leaving the building is so problematic, then outside appointments must be kept at a minimum. When no precipitant can be identified, it is important that staff remain calm and intervene to defuse the problem, whether by distracting the resident, reassuring the resident, or actually removing him or her from the situation. Catastrophic reactions may be less prevalent in special care units, where a dementia-friendly milieu has been created and noxious stimuli and stressors are filtered out as much as is practicable.

The Environmental Context of Symptoms

Behavioral disturbances have a multifactorial derivation, composed of biomedical, emotional, social, and environmental components (Jackson, Spector, & Rabins, 1993). Not all symptoms are problems in all settings. Wandering is a good example. It is problematic on a unit where there are frail patients with walkers or wheelchairs and active corridors replete with supply carts, medication carts, and other equipment. In this setting, a wanderer could be a danger to him- or herself with so many obstacles to overcome and to the other frail patients who could be knocked over if they are in the wanderer's path. On the other hand, in a unit with safe, barrier-free space where all the patients are mobile, walking about, no matter how incessantly, is not a problem behavior.

Other symptoms may also be transformed into purposeful activities by modifying the environment. Rummaging is another example. Going through other residents' belongings and moving and hoarding things is a bothersome behavior on many units. Some facilities, however, have created rummaging areas where residents can go through designated specially stocked drawers and cabinets, try on clothing and accessories, play with dials and knobs, or otherwise channel their energy into an activity that does not inconvenience other residents.

Depression and Dementia

Depression, often occuring together with dementia, is the second most prevalent psychiatric diagnosis in the nursing home, affecting almost one fifth of residents (Katz, Lesher, Kleban, Jethandani, & Parmelee, 1989). Consistent with findings regarding the elderly in a variety of settings, the rates of recognition and treatment of depression are low. Symptoms of depression include sadness, crying, weight loss, slowing down, social withdrawal, loss of motivation, expressions of worthlessness or hopelessness, and sleep difficulties. Depression often is associated with physical illness. It contributes to functional incapacity and diminution of the quality of life of the patient and the caregiver (Teri & Gallagher-Thompson, 1991). Because dementia is prevalent among nursing home residents, the differential diagnosis may be problematic. Depression can coexist with dementia; it is estimated that about 30% of Alzheimer's patients have major depression and even a larger proportion have depressive symptoms (Teri & Reifler, 1987). Depression may cause an overlay of "excess disability" on the already diminished function of individuals with dementia. When the depression is treated, functioning may improve somewhat, but symptoms of dementia remain. The distinctions between depression and dementia are not clear-cut, because the two syndromes have overlapping symptoms. For example, persons with either condition may exhibit a lack of motivation, lack of ability to concentrate or a shortened attention span, and/or sleep-wake disturbances. Psychiatric diagnostic criteria exclude diagnosis of depression in the presence of cognitive impairment. In one study, it was found that 86% of a sample of individuals with dementia had enough "depressive symptoms" so that they would have met DSM-III[1] criteria for depression had they not been cognitively impaired (Merriam, Aronson, Gaston, Wey, & Katz, 1988). The distinctions are further clouded by the diagnostic category of depressive "pseudodementia," which applies to previously nondemented depressed individuals whose cognitive symptoms disappear with treatment of depression. The existence of this syndrome has been called into question by follow-up studies suggesting a disproportionately high incidence of dementia in the pseudodemented after at least one year of follow-up. These other findings raise the possibility of depression as a prodromal state for dementia. Depression can be treated by both pharmacologic and nonpharmacologic interventions.

Dementia Care in the Nursing Home

Defining the care needed by individuals with dementia has been a challenge for the long-term care industry and the reimbursement systems. Disruptive behaviors are a common phenomenon in demented nursing home residents and are intermittent and unpredictable. The agitation and resistance interfere with safety and manageability and increase the nursing staff effort required to care for residents with dementia (Aronson, Cox, Guastadisegni, Frazier, Sherlock, et al., 1992). Yet residents with mild to moderate cognitive impairment who are most disturbed and resistant are usually more ambulatory and less physically disabled than are those patients with severe medical illness. The nursing interventions required are not predominantly physical but involve ongoing supervision, assistance, and prompting. Unlike direct hands-on care and skilled interventions such as injections and dressings, which are administered on a set schedule, the indirect, non-physical interventions for dementia are often done ad hoc and therefore are difficult to document and quantify. Nonetheless, the amount and intensity of nursing staff involvement in performing behavioral interventions equal or may exceed that involved in providing physical assistance.

Management of Behavioral Problems: General Principles

- Management of the dementia patient requires an interdisciplinary team approach. Dementia is a neurological disease with behavioral manifestations that are influenced by environmental and psychosocial variables.
- Comprehensive multidisciplinary assessment is important and should include accurate diagnosis; delineation of the patterns and possible precipitants; assessment of health changes, such as pain or decrements in vision or hearing, or depression, which may impact behavior; review of medication regimen for potential side effects and drug interactions; and psychologic, psychiatric, and/or neurologic consultation as needed.

- Identification of target behaviors for intervention is essential. Expectations must be realistic. Certain behaviors may be annoying but not necessarily in need of, or amenable to, intervention. Repetitive questioning may fall into this category.

- Establishment of an individualized written care plan, including identification of goals, time frames, and interventions is important. For example, is the problem expected to be eliminated entirely or decreased by 50%? In what time frame? What are the roles of the team members in the planned interventions?

- Good communication among staff on all shifts is needed. Individuals with dementia require a *consistent* approach.

- Development of a procedure for monitoring of progress and re-assessment of treatment needs must be in place. Dementing illness is progressive and symptom constellations vary over time, necessitating modification of care plans.

Nonpharmacologic Interventions

The key to most nonpharmacologic interventions resides in appropriate, timely interventions by well-trained staff. Patients who are confused and who lack memory and impulse control need defined boundaries because they cannot recognize danger in their environment and because they are often anxious and insecure. Demented residents require staff vigilance to anticipate problems and intervene before difficulties arise. *Anticipatory management* involves constant supervision and intervention as necessary, for example, redirecting a resident who is lost in a room or a corridor, avoiding a collision between two pacing residents, or removing an obstacle to prevent a fall. At times, staff must also deal with situations they would not have anticipated because of the variability and unpredictability of individuals with dementia.

Residents with dementia have decreased abilities to perform even the simplest activities of daily living and require assistance with task completion in activities such as bathing, dressing, and grooming. Although they may not need to be dressed totally, they may require assistance in terms of selection of clothes and provision of simple directions and single tasks. Dividing an activity into single steps or tasks, which can be mastered by the patient one at a time, is a type of assistance that is called *task segmentation.* Giving the patient one item of clothing at a time to put on, such as a sock or a shirt, and not providing another until the previous task is completed is an example. *Cuing,* that is, providing enough prompts to complete a task or situation, is an adjunctive strategy that is used with dementia patients. The amount of time spent by the nursing aide who assists the resident with dressing may actually be longer than that which would have been spent dressing him or her totally. However, allowing the resident to do as much as possible and retain a sense of autonomy and dignity are important goals for staff interventions as well.

The strategies that work well when residents are cooperative may fail when these same residents are resistant to care. At these times they may be verbally or even physically abusive toward the staff who are trying to help them. In such situations, other strategies must be brought into play—for example, distraction, humor, and/or coaxing. Redirecting or laughing with a resident may avoid a catastrophic reaction.

Staff must learn to be flexible. On a moment's notice, they must be able to step back and redirect their efforts. This may mean deciding to postpone the scheduled bath for a resistive resident or switching from a quiet activity to an active one when residents are agitated.

Redeployment of Resources

Various strategies have been used to improve behavioral management in nursing homes. These include special care units, neurobehavioral units, specialized activities programming such as in-house day care, behavioral consultation teams, staff support groups, and enhanced staff training.

Special care units are often characterized by redeployment of resources for management of dementia-associated behaviors. In addition to environmental modifications that are present in many of these units and staff with special training, these units often have enriched staffing, in terms of a higher ratio of staff to patients and in terms of availability of mental health professionals and activities staff. Furthermore, these units generally incorporate family members as part of the team. Despite the attributes delineated, special care units vary widely on the characteristics that make them "special" and in their philosophies and practice patterns.

Behavioral units are a strategy for management of otherwise hard to place, difficult to manage, behaviorally disturbed patients. The units involve special adaptations for aggressive acting-out patients such as locked doors, and have staff with mental health experience and expertise. These units generally require regulatory waivers and funding exceptions, and few are in existence. These units require close ties with hospital-based geriatric psychiatry programs for diagnostic and pharmacologic support. In these programs, supportive interventions are needed for staff in order to prevent burnout.

Some facilities have behavioral consultation teams to assist staff with difficult patients. These teams may consist of nursing home personnel, outside consultants, such as from a community mental health center, or a combination of both. Disciplines that may be included are psychiatry, psychology, advanced nursing (either geriatric nurse-practitioners or psychiatric nurse-specialists/clinicians), clinical social work, and occupational therapy.

Certain facilities and programs have incorporated staff support groups to provide ongoing emotional support and training. These groups may be led by a staff member or by an outside consultant. An outsider with whom staff can be open without fear of recriminations would be the most appropriate leader. This activity requires an economic commitment by administration in terms of payment for the leader and allocation of staff time to attend these groups.

Enhanced staff training is a hallmark of all good dementia programming and is a component that is easily incorporated into any setting. However, it requires a philosophical and financial commitment on the part of administration to ensure its success. Effective training must include not only line personnel but supervisory leadership. On a continuum of strategies, training is probably the easiest to implement and is, in fact, the most universally effective intervention, not only in terms of impact on patients but also in terms of reduction of staff frustration, burnout, and turnover.

Pharmacologic Interventions

The Omnibus Budget Reconciliation Act of 1987 (OBRA) required that psychotropic medications not be used in place of care, that is, as chemical restraints. Neuroleptics, benzodiazepines, and hypnotic medications are the major categories of drugs used for sedation and anxiety reduction. Demented residents were often medicated with these compounds and physically restrained for "safety purposes," for example, to assure that they would not fall while agitated or wandering, or, in other cases, to assure that they would not wander when there were insufficient staff to provide care. Therefore, these patients were the major beneficiaries of the restraint reduction mandates. Less medication was found to have a positive impact, resulting in less incontinence, less deconditioning, and less skin breakdown, all of which had been increased by iatrogenic, sedation-related immobility. Although actual numbers of falls may have increased slightly, the number of significant injuries did not increase in post-OBRA studies. The decision to allow the patients to have more mobility, even though they may experience more falls, has been referred to as "therapeutic risk taking." The benefits of decreased sedation, increased freedom, and more dignity have far outweighed the alleged risks of injury from falling.

Parenthetically, the use of antidepressant medications remained unchanged post-OBRA. It is firmly believed that this class of drugs is still *underutilized* in nursing homes. This underutilization is multifactorial and related to variables including the confounds to the diagnosis of depression in very sick, very old, often demented individuals; the lack of availability of mental health professionals in nursing homes; misunderstanding of the OBRA regulations, which do not preclude *necessary* drug use; and therapeutic nihilism of many health professionals. Pharmacologic treatment is an important component of many care plans, but is not a substitute for nonpharmacologic approaches to comprehensive management, including environmental adaptations and behavioral interventions.

Summary

The nature of the nursing home population has changed over the past few decades, with a shift away from the medically sick to individuals with neuropsychiatric illness (Rovner & Katz, in press). The type of care provided has not been modified accordingly. Although nursing home patients require both physical assistance and behavioral interventions, the care is skewed toward the physical side. Nursing home patients, despite their myriad of mental health problems, have little or no contact with mental health professionals. Furthermore, the staff who care for them have a paucity of training regarding management of dementia and other neurobehavioral and psychiatric illness. Thus, many patients' psychosocial needs are unmet, and the quality of their lives is impacted negatively.

Revising the nature of nursing home care so that it is congruent with its populace will require increased knowledge by policymakers, regulators, and facilities staff about neurobehavioral conditions and psychiatric illness and their treatment, as well as the management of physical illness and impairments. Research findings need to be disseminated and integrated into practice. In addition, philosophical and financial commitments will be required to effect the systemic changes needed, including new models of care and levels of reimbursement consistent with comprehensive care needs.

Note

1. DSM-III refers to the *Diagnostic and Statistical Manual* of the American Psychiatric Association, Washington, DC.

References

Aronson, M. K., Cox, D., Guastadisegni, P., Frazier, C., Sherlock, L., et al. (1992). Dementia and the nursing home: associated care needs. *Journal of the American Geriatrics Society, 40,* 27-33.

Cohen, D., Eisdrofer, C., Gorelick, P., Paveza, G., Luchins, D. J., et al. (1993). Psychopathology associated with Alzheimer's disease and related disorders. *Journal of Gerontology: Medical Sciences, 48,* M255-M265.

Eisdorfer, C., Cohen, D., Pareza, G., Ashford, W., Luchins, D., et al. (1992). An empirical evaluation of the global deterioration scale for staging Alzheimer's disease. *American Journal of Psychiatry, 149,* 190-194.

Jackson, M. E., Drugovich, M. L., Fretwell, M. D., Spector, W. D. Sternberg, J., & Rosenstein, R. B. (1989). Prevalence and correlates of disruptive behaviors in the nursing home. *Journal of Aging and Health, 1*(3), 349-369.

Jackson, M. E., Spector, W., & Rabins, P. (1993). Risk of behavior problems among U.S. nursing and personal care home residents. *Gerontologist, 33*(1), 193.

Katz, I. R., Lesher, E., Kleban, Jethandani, V. & Parmelee, P. (1989). Clinical features of depression in the nursing home. *International psychogeriatrics, 1,* 5-15.

Merriam, A., Aronson, M. K., Gaston, P., Wey, S., & Katz, I. (1988). The psychiatric symptoms of Alzheimer's disease. *Journal of the American Geriatrics Society, 36,* 7-12.

Rovner, B. W., German, P. S., Broadhead, J., Morriss, R. K., Grant, L.J., et al., (1990). The prevalence and management of dementia and other psychiatric disorders in nursing home. *International Psychogeriatrics, 2,* 13-24.

Rovner, B. W., & Katz, I. R. (in press). Neuropsychiatry in nursing homes. In C. Edward Coffey & Jeffrey L. Cummings (Eds.), *Textbook of geriatric neuropsychiatry.* Washington, DC: APA Press.

Teri, L., & Gallagher-Thompson, D. (1991). Cognitive-behavioral interventions for treatment of depression in Alzheimer's patients. *Gerontologist, 31*(3), 413-416.

Teri, L., Larson, E. L., & Reifler, B.W. (1992). Behavioral disturbances in dementia of the Alzheimer's type. *Journal of the American Geriatrics Society, 36,* 1-6.

Teri, L., & Reifler, B. V. (1987). Depression and dementia. In L. Carstensen & B. Edelstein (Eds.), *Handbook of clinical gerontology* (pp. 112-119). New York: Pergamon.

Zimmer, J. G., Watson, N., & Treat, A. (1984). Behavioral problems among patients in skilled nursing facilities. *American Journal of Public Health 74,* 1118-1121.

8

The Reduction of Restraint Use in the Nursing Home

Donna Cox Post

Patricia Krasnausky

Helene D. Grossman

Deborah Lynch

OBRA: Background and Impact

Over the years nursing homes have evolved from almshouses to mom-and-pop operations to a highly regulated long-term care system. Care in nursing homes has often been scrutinized and criticized. In 1986 the Institute of Medicine appointed a Committee on Nursing Home Regulation to recommend ways to improve nursing home care. From their report evolved the Omnibus Budget Reconciliation Act of 1987 (OBRA 87), which addressed regulatory standards for skilled nursing facilities with a strong emphasis on residents' rights. A major concern was the inappropriate use of restraints. According to OBRA 87, which has been the basis for regulatory change, residents have the right "to be free from physical or mental abuse, corporal punishment, involuntary seclusion, and any physical or chemical restraints imposed for purposes of discipline or convenience and not required to treat the resident's medical symptoms" (p. 165).

This statement illustrates the change in focus brought about by OBRA 87 as compared to prior regulations. Previously, quality care focused on nursing home structure and environment rather than on the residents. This perspective is based on the regulatory history of the nursing home itself. Regulations for nursing homes were promulgated by the federal government for facility participation in the Medicare and Medicaid reimbursement programs. These regulations focused on the bare necessities, such as staffing requirements, services of an RN and charge nurse, along with standards related to fire safety, medical supervision, drug dispensing, dietary matters, and sanitation (Waldman, 1985). If the nursing home complied with the mandated conditions, it was then assumed that the residents were receiving quality care.

Accepted practice for caring for frail elderly nursing home residents was directed toward resident safety to avoid unattended wandering, falls, broken hips, and fear of long hospital stays. As society became more litigious, the perceived threat of malpractice suits prevailed. Facilities sought to protect residents, to give them a safe place, and to evolve standards of care that included the use of restraints, both chemical and physical. The pharmaceutical industry made drugs available that quieted the disturbed and agitated resident. Industry provided physical restraints to limit the movement of residents.

OBRA 87 shifted the emphasis to quality of life and resident choice, with an increased focus on the resident condition and experience within the care process (Ammentorp, Gossett, & Poe, 1991). A quality experience involves freedom from restraint, unless the resident presents a clear and present danger to self or others.

Rationale for Restraint Use

The new regulations were predicated on the belief that in the past, use of restraints in some nursing homes were imposed primarily for staff convenience rather than the safety of the patient. In 1977 Covert, Rodrigues, and Solomon, all geropsychiatric consultants to nursing homes, reported that in their experience "chemical and mechanical restraints have become widely used as a convenient substitute for adequate supervision and treatment, and have thus become a silent but potent partner in accomplishing the warehousing of human beings" (p. 86).

In a comprehensive review, Evans and Strumpf (1989) reported that use of restraints systematically increased in relation to the patient's age and level of cognitive impairment. Residents who screamed, wandered, or were socially disruptive were especially likely to be restrained. They cited other studies indicating that the most common reason for use of restraints cited by staff members was to protect the patient or others, followed by a means to control behavior; however, other reasons included "insufficient staffing, staff attitudes, administrative pressures to avoid possible litigation, or normative values."

The Paradoxical Effect of Restraints

What has become a well-known paradox in the literature on use of restraints is that the restraints themselves often serve to exacerbate the very behaviors they were meant to control. According to Collopy, Boyle, and Jennings (1991),

> Far from protecting patients from harm, restraints inflict it. Physical risks include bed sores, infections, reduced circulation, muscle weakness, pneumonia, loss of appetite and incontinence caused by immobility. . . . Psychological risks, more difficult to quantify, include humiliation, fear of abandonment, impairment of self-image, agitation, panic and disorientation. (p. 11)

Understanding "Problem" Behaviors

Based on the problems associated with the use of restraints, Moss and La Puma (1991) cautioned that restraints should be considered an "investigational or nonvalidated therapy" (p. 23). Rather than using restraints, a more productive approach is to examine alternative methods based on an understanding of the problem behaviors (Collopy, Boyle, & Jennings, 1991). This approach recognizes that problem behaviors, such as wandering or screaming, may actually be the residents' response to a new environment, a medical problem, or attempts at communication.

An example cited by Covert, Rodrigues, and Solomon (1977) concerned an 85-year-old nursing home resident who had severe dementia and was found on the floor, probably the result of falling out of bed. To prevent this from happening again, the woman was restrained in bed. She began to scream and became quite agitated, which resulted in further application of physical and chemical restraints. This continued for several weeks, until a psychiatric consultant was called in, who simply asked the woman if she had any pain. The woman answered yes, and after a physical evaluation, it was discovered that she had a femoral neck fracture suffered in the original fall. After the fracture was treated, the woman returned to her original calm state.

Based on such cases, Covert, Rodrigues, and Solomon (1977) recommended that, except in emergencies, restraints should be ordered by a physician only after personally examining the resident's physical and mental status and that these orders should never be part of a routine standing order. In addition, "problem behaviors" may be problems only in certain contexts. For example, wandering is not a problem in a wandering unit.

Programs Aimed at Reducing the Use of Physical Restraints

Recognizing that the use of physical restraints can violate both the health and dignity of residents, several long-term care facilities embarked on programs of restraint reduction. Some of these programs were initiated to reduce and remove restraints prior to OBRA, with emphasis on promoting resident freedom and dignity as well as providing an environment that encourages safety and autonomy.

The use of physical restraints had become a standard intervention within many long-term care settings. When New York State developed its funding initiative for nursing home care innovations/research regarding dementia, the issue of restraint use was a priority area. Several awards were made, and the following information is based on these early demonstrations. The demonstration facilities sought to challenge the notion that restraints prevent injury. With an emphasis on exploring alternatives and monitoring responses, the facilities demonstrated the feasibility of a "restraint-free environment."

Program Development

Education was an integral component of the successful implementation of the demonstration programs. The educational programs focused on ethical and philosophical considerations, benefits, risks, alternative methods, legal aspects, and statistical information. Individual staff members had to be convinced that restraints were not necessary and that there was a need to change previous practices, habits, and beliefs. Board, administrative, and medical staff support and encouragement were sought and received at the initiation of the projects. Additionally, educational programs were held for the families and responsible parties of the residents in order to introduce the new policy.

Program Initiation

Although the exact sequence may have varied from facility to facility, generally on completion of the educational programs, individual nursing units were selected to initiate the new program. The units with staff most positive toward the concept of restraint removal served as the demonstration units for subsequent facilitywide implementation.

All residents with restraints were selected for program inclusion, with an initial focus on the easier cases. The removal of restraints from the residents required carefully formulated individualized care plans. Staff assessed the residents and the reasons that had necessitated the initial use of restraints; strategies were then developed to remove the restraints.

Alternatives to Restraints

It was recognized that in providing alternatives it was important to manipulate the environment and *not* the resident, because demented residents usually cannot learn new information. The following is a description of environmental manipulations that were accomplished at one or more facilities participating in early demonstrations.

Alarm systems. An alarm system was installed at one large facility where several doors to each unit presented a problem in caring for the wandering resident. A transmitter worn on the ankle of the preidentified residents triggered the alarm and alerted staff when residents attempted to exit the unit. The system enabled the staff to monitor resident activity and allowed the resident freedom of movement. Additional alarms were installed on exterior doors to form a dual system. Today many facilities have some type of alarm system, whether or not they have a specialized dementia unit.

Barrier between units. Another concern was developing a device to limit the wandering of residents between areas. One facility used a detachable plastic strip that acted as a barrier between two nursing units. A 2-inch strip was attached with Velcro® at midchest level across the doorway to the adjoining nursing unit. This strip redirected the residents' wandering, yet allowed staff to move freely between units. Similar strips were used at other internal doors to deter wandering residents from specific areas. Environmental cues used by other facilities included stop signs, traffic lights, and camouflaging the doors with murals.

Bed alarms. Bed alarms were utilized to assist in monitoring residents who tended to climb out of bed at night. A sensor placed under the sheets was attached to an alarm positioned on the bed frame. The system proved overly sensitive and sounded when a resident turned from side to side. This was particularly true when the resident was light in weight. Therefore, in that facility the bed alarm was used as an alternative to physical restraints only when a resident could not be otherwise monitored. These bed alarms can help to limit the use of bed rails at night.

"Special" chairs. Armchairs were modified to increase the backward tilt of the seat, thereby increasing the time needed for a resident to rise from the chair. This increase in time allowed nursing staff to respond and assist or ambulate the residents as needed. The chair has been effective for those residents who have been restrained because of unsteady gait. This chair resembles the old-fashioned porch chairs or Adirondack chairs. It is most successfully utilized during the first 2 to 3 days after restraints are removed.

Central supervision. Congregating residents in a central location for better supervision and activities programming was found to be essential in one demonstration project. Staff was assigned to the central location for 30-minute shifts to improve the safety of residents who were no longer restrained.

Program Outcomes

The restraint reduction projects met with great success at the demonstration facilities. They showed that dramatic changes can be made when a total institutionwide commitment and belief exist that restraints are not compatible with quality care or quality of life. Operating without restraints became an essential part of the culture of these institutions. In most of these facilities, use of restraints was reduced to less than 5% of their population. Restraints are used as a last resort, are the least restrictive type, and are used for an absolute minimum period of time. Alternatives to restraint are explored on an ongoing basis. With the nonuse of restraints, adverse effects are prevented and resident dignity is preserved while safety and security are maintained. With OBRA regulations, limitation of restraint use is no longer optional but required.

Throughout the duration of the respective programs, the number of falls and injuries were monitored. Falls continued to be a concern, and it was difficult to find a causal relationship between restraint release and falls because they continued to occur both among these residents who had been restrained and among those who had never been restrained. Some previously restrained residents did not fall at all. Overall, injuries did not increase.

Reducing Chemical Restraints

As efforts in some facilities were focused on reducing physical restraints, others initiated programs to modify patterns of prescribing psychotropic drugs for the elderly. The high rate of psychotropic prescriptions (often approaching 50% of the population) caused concern for the quality and appropriateness of these orders in long-term care facilities.

In the majority of interventions to change prescribing patterns, most efforts have focused on physician education. The results have been promising, but often minimal and temporary. Insofar as prescribing practices in the nursing facility are a result of many factors, attempts that do not involve the support, education, and awareness of other personnel, particularly nursing, are of very limited value. A multidisciplinary, multifaceted strategy, as implemented in one nursing home, exemplifies a more successful approach.

Program Implementation

The program initiative included a psychosocial team to coordinate all psychiatric services, the introduction of staff development programs to teach behavioral management techniques, and formal psychopharmacologic education and physician consultation. A psychiatric social worker directed the psychosocial team. Weekly meetings were held and staff from all clinical disciplines, including pastoral counseling, dietary, housekeeping, and administration, were encouraged to participate in meetings as well.

In-service education and staff development programs were used to introduce new policies and to facilitate changes in staff behavior. Monthly lectures for the nursing staff focused on the appropriate use of psychotropic medications as well as behaviorally oriented alternatives. The program targeted specific symptoms as indicators for psychotropic drugs and the notation of specific therapeutic goals in the record. Alternatives to psychotropic medication were illustrated and included increased activity during the day, short-term addition of one-to-one contact, reduction in caffeine, and removal of sensory impediments through provision of hearing and vision aids. A physician conducted the educational sessions with brief, graphic educational materials clearly showing the choice of preferred agents, with indications and contraindications. Nursing educators provided a series of conferences for nursing assistants, with an ongoing dialogue about patient behavior, symptoms, and skills needed to cope with demanding and disruptive residents.

Staff development programs included eight weekly multidisciplinary sessions of 3 hours each in which a geriatric nurse-educator led an experiential group process designed to encourage a team-oriented care strategy and to build empathy in caregivers. Increasing resident activity through the use of a designated room with trained staff to engage disruptive dementia residents in tasks was also demonstrated. Medications were not used to deal with episodes of agitation. Instead, disruptive outbursts were behaviorally modified during the group.

Psychiatric and psychopharmacologic consultations were made readily available. The weekly psychosocial team meetings and the ongoing in-service education programs opened a forum to discuss resident problems as well as staff difficulties with new situations.

The in-service education programs did not directly involve the unit attending physicians. However, the psychiatrist provided weekly memos written to individual physicians with recommendations for modifying medication use and reinforcement of desired changes. Formal consultation requests as well as ad hoc, informal contacts with the primary physicians allowed the advancement of appropriate psychopharmacology for the residents.

Results

Overall there was a 32% reduction across all classes of psychotropics over a 12-month period. Antipsychotic agents were decreased by 31% and anti-anxiety agents by 17%, while the use of antidepressants increased by 19%. The use of antihistamines, often tried to induce sleep in the elderly, declined by 86%.

Polypharmacy, that is, use of several agents simultaneously, was also substantially reduced over the 12-month period, with a trend toward single agent therapy. At the outset, 30 residents were receiving two or more psychotropics, and at the study's end, only 10 were on this regimen.

Before the program was initiated, physical restraints were ordered for 36% of the residents; this declined substantially over the 12 months. The number of falls reported remained consistent throughout the observation period.

The intervention differed from others in that formal education regarding the appropriate use of psychotropics was focused on the nursing staff. In nursing facilities, nurses are the major providers of day-to-day resident care, as well as the principal identifiers of emerging patient problems. The nurses' pivotal role must be incorporated in any effort to implement new treatment strategies.

The results demonstrated that an aggressive in-service education program for staff, the use of "academic" case conferences, and the illustration of behavioral and social alternatives to medication can substantially reduce the use and improve the choice of psychotropics. Also, the reduction in psychotropics was accompanied by an increase in the number and daily doses of antidepressants. Depression is prevalent, but often neglected and undermedicated among nursing home residents (Lantz, Louis, Lowenstein, & Kennedy, 1990).

This program suggests that a multidisciplinary, multifaceted approach can reduce the use of medications for psychosis, anxiety, and sleep; increase the more appropriate use of antidepressants; and introduce alternative methods of treatment in the nursing home. Physical restraints were not substituted for psychotropics and frequent falls due to agitation from medication withdrawal did not occur. Although it was the impression of involved staff that the mental health of the residents was improved by these interventions, there are no data beyond these clinical impressions as to symptom reduction or functional improvement. Thus, research is needed in the nursing home to measure the impact of the reduction of medications on residents' psychosocial well-being. Table 8.1 summarizes possible variables that may be measured in the monitoring of the use of restraints—whether physical or chemical—within a given facility.

Regulatory/Legal Issues

Practice innovations, along with the regulations implemented under OBRA 87, "clearly and intentionally tilt the regulatory odds against the provider who indiscriminately applies physical restraints" (Kapp, 1990, p. 4). The reason for this is that the "legal standard of care" is decided, in part, by the customary practice of the industry at the time a lawsuit is filed. Due to the legislation, the mounting evidence that restraints may actually do more harm than good, and the success of less restrictive environmental and behavioral interventions, the standard of care has shifted toward a restraint-free environ-

TABLE 8.1 Considerations for Monitoring Restraint Use

Number of residents physically restrained

Number of residents chemically restrained

Number of residents physically and chemically restrained

Number of "emergency" restraint orders

Documented reasons for these interventions and frequency of reassessment

Documentation of attempts at alternative interventions

Types of restraints

Duration of usage

Adverse effects noted

Rate of falls/injuries

Changes in ADL status

Activities participation

Changes in mood

Changes in mental status

Resident and/or family satisfaction

ment. This shift will make it easier for nursing homes to justify nonuse of restraints and conversely make it more difficult to justify use of restraints (Kapp, 1990).

Issues in Risk Management

Basically, the issue of the use of restraints in the nursing home is an issue of risk management. At the present time, increased risk is associated with improper use of restraints rather than in the failure to restrain a resident. Recent research

(Kellogg, 1993) has demonstrated that the use of physical restraints is associated with both increased death and disease rates and that restraint use does not reduce serious falls and their associated complications.

OBRA has had the desired impact, that is, the reduction of the utilization of physical and chemical restraints; however, in some circumstances the use of restraints may be the only way to protect a resident from injuring her- or himself or others. The following guidelines are suggested:

- Facility policies and procedures that address the requirements of OBRA 1987 regulations in the use of physical and chemical restraints must be developed and communicated to caregivers, residents, and families.
- Education for physicians in the area of geriatrics in general and the appropriate use of restraints in particular is essential for medical practice in the nursing home.
- In-service programs should be ongoing for all staff to educate them on the appropriate use of restraints, along with the alternative methods available. An emphasis should be placed on the use of positive behavioral management techniques and environmental manipulations.
- Restraints should not be used routinely because there is no evidence to validate their use. Rather, there must be a physician's order pertinent to the specific situation.
- Consent must be obtained from the resident or the family with regard to use of restraints, and the benefits and risks associated with their use must be explained.
- When there exists no alternative to the use of restraints, the least restrictive restraint should be ordered by a physician for a specified time period, with frequent checks for proper application and resident comfort. In addition, restraints require release every 2 hours for exercise and toileting.
- In emergency situations, restraints may be applied without consent, but for a very limited period and under very specific conditions.
- When chemical restraints are to be used, the lowest effective dose of medication is to be used for a specified period of time and dosage reductions are to be tried in determining the lowest possible clinically effective dosage.

TABLE 8.2 Summary Principles Regarding Restraint Use

Allow the residents as much autonomy and dignity as possible in order to maximize their remaining capacities.

It is important to manipulate the environment and modify staff behaviors as demented residents cannot learn new things.

Although care planning involves assessment of the resident in the context of his or her environment, behavioral interventions require that identification be made of the target behaviors that require modification and efforts be directed accordingly.

Less is more. The fewer the restraints, chemical or physical, the better, because restraints may add to the confusion and frustration of demented residents. However, in cases where psychotropic drugs are necessary, they must be used effectively and appropriately.

- Monitoring of impact and potential side effects of certain psychotropic drugs (neuroleptics) is now a requirement. Certain other drugs may not be used under any circumstances.
- The prevalence of restraint use must be audited and monitored by quality assurance, and modifications must be made by the care team as problems are identified.

In summary, appropriate restraint use in the nursing home is an integral part of quality of care and quality of life. It requires careful assessment and monitoring as well as ongoing resident, staff, and family communication and orientation. Due to the heterogeneity of residents and facilities, general recommendations must be implemented on a case-by-case basis. Table 8.2 lists some summary principles.

References

Ammentorp, W., Gossett, K. D., & Poe, E. N. (1991). *Quality assurance for long-term care providers.* Newbury Park, CA: Sage.

Collopy, B., Boyle, P., & Jennings, B. (1991). New directions in nursing home ethics. *Hastings Center Report,* Special Supplement March-April, 1-15.

Covert, A. B., Rodrigues, T., & Solomon, K. (1977). The use of mechanical and chemical restraints in nursing homes. *Journal of the American Geriatrics Society, 25*(2), 85-89.

Evans, L. K., & Strumpf, N. E. (1989). Tying down the elderly: A review of the literature on physical restraint. *Journal of the American Geriatrics Society, 37,* 65-74.

Kapp, M. B. (1990). *Legal liability implications of nursing home restraints.* Unpublished essay, Wright State University School of Medicine, Office of Geriatric Medicine and Gerontology, Dayton, OH.

Kellogg, K. (1993). Restraining nursing home residents is costly procedure. *News and Information Service, The University Record* [Newsletter]. Ann Arbor: University of Michigan.

Lantz, M. S., Louis, A., Lowenstein, G., & Kennedy, G. J. (1990). A longitudinal study of psychotropic prescriptions in a teaching nursing home. *American Journal of Psychiatry, 147*(12), 1637-1639.

Moss, R. J., & La Puma, J. (1991). The ethics of mechanical restraints. *Hastings Center Report, 21*(1), 22-25.

Omnibus Budget Reconciliation Act of 1987 (OBRA). Public Law 100-203. December 22, 1987.

Waldman, S. (1985). A legislative history of nursing home care. In R. J. Vogel & H. C. Palmer (Eds.), *Long-term care: Perspectives from research and demonstrations.* Rockville, MD: Aspen.

9

Staffing Patterns and Training for Competent Dementia Care

Cynthia Frazier
Lila Sherlock

Staffing is a critical factor in the successful functioning of nursing facilities that provide care for dementia patients, regardless of whether the residents are grouped in specialized units or distributed throughout the facility. Staffing is a critical factor in the successful functioning of any facility. A multidisciplinary group of staff (including nursing, social work, and therapy) are needed to provide dignified care.

Traditionally, however, reimbursement for long-term care facilities has been dependent on patients' "skilled nursing" needs, with those having the sickest patients getting more resources—a pattern derived from the practices of the acute hospital. This weighting of reimbursement was designed to encourage long-term care facilities to admit a greater number of medically ill patients, rather than having them remain in expensive hospital beds once their acute illness passed. With the incentives provided by New York State's Resource Utilization Groups (RUG) system of reimbursement, that is, higher rates for greater acuity, facilities could hire sufficient nursing staff to deal with increased medical needs. A consequence of this policy was to penalize institutions that serve individuals with dementing illnesses who are otherwise healthy.

In fact, those who care for dementia patients are aware that the level of effort required to manage the activities of daily living (ADL) for such persons exceeds that which is necessary for those who are more cognitively intact (Aronson, Cox, & Guastadisegni, 1992). Interventions that encourage independence and prevent severe behavioral problems are much more time-consuming than those that involve straightforward physical care. To accomplish this, staff training in management of dementia symptoms must be ongoing. Staff must also be supported in their efforts to deal creatively with patients whose behavior problems are unpredictable and intermittent and who often respond differently to the same intervention. The challenge of providing competent care for dementia patients is enormous.

Selection of Staff

Caring for demented individuals is very staff intensive. If given the opportunity, it is advisable, therefore, to select staff to maximize the fit between the job requirements and the personality of the employee. At Morningside Nursing Home located in New York City, an interview[1] was designed to facilitate this. The criteria used are included in Table 9.1.

During the interview, the interviewer poses 15 questions with subparts corresponding to the nine criteria (see Appendix). The candidate is rated on each criterion (rating scale also contained in the appendix). Thus, prospective employees can be rated objectively and compared with one another. This process may be useful for justifying employee selection in facilities with labor contracts.

TABLE 9.1 Criteria for Working With Patients With Dementia

Personal warmth
Communication skills with residents; family members; other staff members
Past experience working with dementia, groups
Knowledge of symptomatology/behavioral manifestations of dementia
Ability to work as a team
Initiative/creativity
Receptivity to supervision
Emergency responsiveness
Good attendance on the job

Note: These criteria have not been empirically validated.

Another technique to incorporate in the interview process is to give the candidate a tour of the dementia unit or program and watch for any unsolicited information he or she may reveal such as comfort level, communication style, spontaneity, and so forth. Whenever possible, invite the applicant to participate in some aspect of care to directly observe the candidate's ability to interact with patients. Starting out with motivated staff is a definite advantage.

Flexible, but Not Interchangeable, Staff

A popular concept in management of dementia patients has been "flexible" staff, that is, staff fully trained in all aspects of dementia care so that everyone can respond sensitively to the behavioral manifestations of dementia. The goal is to encourage the development of a therapeutic milieu for the dementia patient in which the environment and the caregiving staff provide a structured and consistent setting in response to patient needs.

When developing staff assignments, it is important to recognize that the traditional division of labor in long-term care facilities cannot be completely disregarded. The hard facts remain: Nursing staff is required to provide daily physical care, and social work and recreation staff, no matter how attuned to resident needs, are rarely involved in the actual toileting, dressing, and feeding of the patients. Similarly, housekeeping, maintenance, and dietary staff have highly regulated functions to perform.

Because nursing assistants have the most interaction with residents on a daily basis, it is necessary for them to learn techniques for the management of behavioral problems. It is also desirable that the importance of their work be recognized and acknowledged by other members of the multidisciplinary team. Team training must address these attitudinal issues as well as the specifics of dementia care. Although staff roles need to be discrete, a unified, coordinated team approach to providing consistent, appropriate care is essential.

Mainstreaming Versus Special Care Units

Although there are a variety of formats for the care of dementia patients in a nursing home, the choice basically comes down to two approaches—mainstreaming or special care units.

Mainstreaming

Mainstreaming has a number of advantages. Apart from avoiding the stigma of a label that often accompanies residing in a dementia unit, mainstreaming is advantageous in facilities where size or other factors prohibit the creation of a separate unit. Patients can reside in any area of a facility and still receive the benefits of special programs. In-house dementia day care and primary nursing are two examples of adaptations that work when patients are mainstreamed.

In-house dementia day care. In-house dementia day care is an example of a program that can be utilized in any setting. Residents with dementia reside in all areas of the facilities but are brought to a central location for periods ranging from a few hours to all day. Specially trained multidisciplinary staff and volunteers assist the patients in programs of music, activities, meals, reminiscence, and sensory awareness that help keep them involved and functioning at their best cognitive level.

Primary nursing. Another approach to management of the dementia patient that can be utilized in most facilities is primary nursing, the permanent assignment of the same staff to the same patients.[2] The rationale for the primary care model is that nursing assistants who care for the same patients on a long-term basis will have knowledge of personal care preferences of residents; have better recall of the resident's family, life history, and communication patterns; develop better rapport with families; be more sensitive to subtle changes in resident functioning; be more alert to skin breakdown; be better able to coordinate care among assigned patients because of familiarity with time requirements for various tasks; and be able to cooperate more efficiently with co-workers in assisting with lifts and transfers. The overriding rationale is the consistency that this approach provides for confused, sometimes unpredictable, and difficult to manage patients.

Nursing assistants who worked with this system preferred it to their previous rotation schedule because it let them know in advance what to expect for the day, gave them a greater sense of control over work, and provided them with an opportunity to build rapport with their patients. Problems with this model included dealing with floating or part-time staff, having to team up with someone they did not like, or having too many very heavy or difficult patients giving them an unbalanced assignment. Primary nursing assistants have reported the need for nursing supervisers to ensure all individuals were "holding up their end of the team."

Dementia consultation team. Another model for providing specialized management of the difficult resident is the dementia consultation team, a multidisciplinary group that assists staff with assessment and problem solving. The team may consist of any combination of psychiatric nurse-clinician, psychiatrist, psychologist, social worker, and occupational or physical therapist. The team may be brought in for consultation and may provide care planning as well as training for all involved unit staff. In some facilities restraint reduction teams may serve this function. In others, a nurse-clinician, psychologist, or psychiatrist may assume these responsibilities.

Special Care Units

Special care units are also believed to have advantages, despite a study (Holmes et al., 1990) that suggested that the cognitive function of individuals in dementia units declined at a rate similar to that of the demented patients in nonspecialized nursing units.

Homogeneity can be viewed as an advantage to special units. Patients can be selected according to their cognitive and behavioral function, and programs can be structured accordingly. It has been reported that special care units provide the best care when the patients in them are most homogeneous in their needs and level of function.

A special unit allows for substantial family involvement. The family's understanding of the disease and progression of dementia and their support of staff efforts is an important factor in building and maintaining an effective patient treatment program.

Another advantage is the potential for rearrangement in staffing patterns. This is important for several reasons. Flexibility in staff hours and duties is extremely useful when dealing with the well-recognized phenomenon of sundowning, the intensity of behavioral symptoms in the late afternoon. With the freedom to schedule some nursing staff to work from 8 a.m. to 4 p.m. and others from 10 a.m. to 6 p.m., it is possible to provide floor coverage during the times when the rest of the staff is engaged in change of shift report or attending to meals and when some patients are most agitated. Having activities staff on hand during these times will keep residents positively involved and active. Inclusion of a nursing assistant in the activity provides continuity and a sense of security for the residents.

Yet another aspect of flexibility is that it allows for enhancing, or increasing, the number of staff on the evening and nighttime shifts. This is a major advantage when caring for individuals in whom sleep-wake cycles are commonly disrupted. Some facilities mobilize all staff and volunteers during mealtimes and other periods of intensive activities, to provide more individualized attention.

Clearly, the size of a facility will affect the type of special unit and the services provided. Caring for demented individuals is a labor-intensive experience, no matter what the format, and this human effort costs money. Because personnel is generally the largest single expenditure in any facility, long-term care facilities are faced with a challenge: how to provide dementia care when reimbursement may not be commensurate with the level of patient need. The goal is to produce a therapeutic environment, not just an environment with therapies. Training is an essential ingredient for accomplishing this.

Training Staff to Work With Demented Patients

Due to the progressive nature of dementia, each demented resident will demonstrate a gradual decline in intellectual functioning and in performance of activities of daily living and will manifest signs of personality disorganization. In addition, idiosyncratic behaviors such as disrobing, hoarding, screaming, and unprovoked verbal and physical aggression will occur frequently and will require individualized interventions.

Burnout

The unpredictable display of "psychiatric" behaviors in demented individuals is difficult for staff. Many employees begin to experience burnout. Burnout may be manifested as physical exhaustion (for example, increased tardiness/absenteeism and an increased frequency of illness and/or accident proneness); emotional exhaustion (e.g., feelings of depletion, depression, hopelessness, or entrapment); or mental exhaustion, such as development of negative attitudes toward self and work, job dissatisfaction, hostility, and interstaff conflict (Pines, Aronson, & Kafry, 1981). Staff members experiencing burnout will impede team functioning. Burnout can be minimized by training staff to better understand dementia and intervene therapeutically and by fostering a team approach.

Specialized Training Techniques

It is vital that all dementia programs provide staff training. Such a training program should be interdisciplinary and include representatives from each department that provides patient services. These departments include nursing, social services, occupational therapy, physical therapy, recreational therapy, dietary services, housekeeping, chaplaincy, security, and volunteers. It is essential to include nursing assistants in dementia training because they spend approximately 90% of work hours directly interacting with residents. The interdisciplinary approach to training fosters a sense of teamwork while simultaneously increasing staff knowledge. The goal of training is to increase the participants' knowledge about dementia and therapeutic intervention. In addition, goals such as heightening a personal sense of confidence, enhancing team communication, and improving problem-solving abilities can be incorporated.

Because this training is generally provided on the job in a nonacademic milieu to adults of varying educational and literacy levels, the training must be developed accordingly. Eight principles of adult learning can be incorporated in the development of a training program (Knowles, 1969).

> ***Principle 1:*** Adults should be involved in the process of self-diagnosis of needs for learning.

Before initiating any type of training, it is wise to directly assess the learning needs of the staff. Of course, it is more likely that staff will reveal areas of knowledge deficit if the trainer is a neutral, nonsupervisory staff member. Also, when allowed to choose areas of learning, staff appear more interested (e.g., ask more questions) and are more challenged by the material (e.g., bring personal anecdotes to discuss). Generally, staff will request that the curriculum include a review of symptomatology associated with dementia. When staff are able to connect aberrant behaviors with the disease process, they are less likely to experience personal ineffectiveness often symptomatic of burnout.

Another area of training often requested is how to manage specific behavior problems. Although there are basic principles for intervening with the demented, there are no techniques that work with every patient or work each time employed. It is more useful, then, to teach staff to assess behavior of each individual from three perspectives: the resident, the staff member, and the situation.[3]

> *Resident:* Does the resident have a mental or physical condition that affects this behavior?
>
> *Staff:* Is the resident reacting to something I am doing or not doing? Can I change something about myself that would help the resident? How do I feel about this resident and this behavior? Do my feelings show?
>
> *Situation:* Is the resident reacting to the situation or something in the environment? What is it? How can I change it?

By taking all three perspectives, a more individualized treatment plan can be developed. It is useful to specify in writing what interventions will be employed (i.e., what to do and what not to do) so that staff providing care at any time (or any shift) can adhere to the plan in a consistent manner. It is also important to stress how staff behavior and feelings can evoke both desired and undesired responses from a resident. As staff begin to recognize this, they will become less defensive and more open to analyzing their own behavior when problem solving. As a result, the staff will experience a sense of effectiveness rather than a sense of futility when attempting to change behaviors caused by an irreversible condition.

When staff members recognize their importance as therapeutic agents, they often will request training about forming therapeutic relationships and about communication techniques. Modules may be developed pertaining to verbal and nonverbal communication, active and passive listening, communicating with touch, communicating with the language-impaired, win-win communication, communication with family members, and written communication (i.e., documentation).

> **Principle 2:** The learning climate most conducive is one that attends to the physical environment and psychological atmosphere.

If possible, it is more conducive to learning to hold training sessions off the unit to minimize disruptions caused by the daily routine. Select a room that is comfortable and well ventilated and provide refreshments to facilitate a relaxed atmosphere. Set parameters for participation that will clarify the expectations of training (e.g., feel free to disagree; ask questions; share your opinions/experiences). Establish a nonjudgmental environment where there are no wrong answers and where all opinions are respected.

> **Principle 3:** Learners should be involved in the process of planning their own learning with the teacher serving as a procedural guide and content resource.

Once the staff have identified their learning needs, the trainer should conduct a planning session with the participants (or representatives) to mutually determine the content and the logistics such as what time, what day, how long, how frequently, and where. In this way, staff resistances may be reduced. Be aware that making decisions as a group will take more time, but will reinforce team communication and cooperation.

> ***Principle 4:*** Greater emphasis can be placed on techniques that tap experience of adult learners such as group techniques, role playing, simulation exercises, skill-practice exercises, demonstration, and action projects.

Adult learners respond better to experiential, rather than didactic, teaching techniques. Training exercises can be developed with case vignettes, role playing, self-assessments, demonstrations, and the like. Films and videos are effective aids to learning. Discussion is probably the most useful method for stimulating active participation. When opinions are respected in an atmosphere where there are no wrong answers nor disciplinary consequences, staff members are more likely to share personal ideas and be open to examining them. Staff behavior will begin to change as new information is synthesized.

> ***Principle 5:*** Emphasis is placed on practical application of learning that includes provision for applying learning in the learners' day-to-day lives.

Behavior change will occur when staff have the opportunity to apply new concepts and methods to the actual work situation. Thus, it is advisable to allot time during each session for the discussion of specific patient problems or situations to foster group problem solving. In addition, meetings can be arranged after the completion of formal training to continue this process.

Principle 6: Evaluation is attained through a process of self-evaluation in which the teacher devotes time and energy to helping adults gather evidence for themselves about progress they are making toward their educational goals.

Exams are not recommended for adult learners participating in an on-the-job training program because tests often evoke performance anxiety and job insecurity. A process of self-evaluation is preferable. In some instances, a test can be self-administered and used as the basis for a group discussion. The staff member may then privately assess how much of the material he or she has comprehended. Another useful method of self-evaluation is case presentation. Using the format of assessing behavior from three perspectives—that of the resident, the staff member, and the situation—any staff member can make an oral presentation at a treatment planning meeting. In this way, a staff member can evaluate his or her own understanding of a patient.

Principle 7: Although adults respond to external motivators (e.g., salary increase), the more potent motivators are internal—self-esteem, recognition, greater self-confidence, and the like.

To be realistic, staff will always ask for salary increases. However, the motivation to continue working with the demented is internally driven by a sense of effectiveness—"I make a difference." Self-esteem, confidence, and job satisfaction are elevated by recognition, which can take the form of a graduation ceremony after completion of training, a certificate of attendance, a pin to wear on one's uniform, or a personal handshake from the administrator. Recognition does not have to be delayed for a special event; rather, it can be given after a therapeutic intervention is made by any staff member. Staff often remark that the most satisfying motivator is an exchange of daily courtesy (e.g., "Thank you!" from a resident or "Good job!" from another staff member).

Principle 8: An organization that fosters adult learning to the fullest degree stimulates individual self-renewal and encourages its personnel to engage in a process of continuous change and growth.

Working with the demented is physically, emotionally, and mentally draining, and burnout is a potential job hazard. As part of the training curriculum, it is important to address the common emotional reactions of staff (e.g., frustration, anger, disappointment, despair, etc.) and how these may be signs of burnout. Staff must feel that assistance is available for dealing with symptoms of burnout without fear of reprisal. Some useful methods include individual counseling, team ventilation sessions, and task or patient reassignment. Balancing a staff member's caseload with lower and higher functioning residents may also be helpful.

Team Building

Training that facilitates team building, whether explicitly or implicitly, helps combat personal burnout and reduces staff turnover. When facility policy encourages staff members to work together, everybody benefits. Team problem solving can validate one's feelings of frustration and impart a sense of collaboration and support, making staff feel more effective and open to change (e.g., new programs, new job tasks, new documentation, etc.).

Conclusion

In summary, there is general agreement that effective staffing is critical to good dementia care. Training is a strong determinant of a quality program. What is clear is that training has a positive impact on the patient, the staff, and the facility.

APPENDIX

Staff Selection Interview

1. Tell me about yourself.
   Your family?
   Your interests/hobbies?
   Your most valuable strength?
   Your most important weakness?

   Criteria:
   Personal warmth
   Communication skills with other staff (interviewer)

2. Tell me about your work history.
   Have your ever worked with people who have dementia?

   Criterion:
   Past experience working with dementia

3. Have you ever been involved in running a therapeutic group? If so, what type?

   Criterion:
   Past experience working with groups

4. Why are you interested in working in a dementia program?
   Why would you like working with a population that is not

going to get better, can't communicate, and is prone to assaultiveness?

Criterion:
Initiative

5. Describe a patient (resident) of yours who you feel was a real problem for you and how you were able to intervene.

Criterion:
Past experience

6. If a family member approaches you about a problem, how would you handle this?

Criteria:
Personal warmth
Communication skills with family member

7. If you disagree with the treatment strategy developed at the team conference, what would you do about it?

Criteria:
Ability to work as a team
Receptivity to supervision
Communication skills with other staff (cohort/supervisors)

8. You are scheduled to assist the recreational therapist in a group, but the recreational therapist calls in sick. What would you do?

Criteria:
Initiative/Creativity
Ability to work as a team

9. How do you communicate with a client who has difficulty making his/her needs known?

Criteria:
Knowledge of dementia
Personal warmth
Past experience working with dementia
Communication skills with resident

10. If a resident who needed a bath refused and became aggressive, what would you do?

Criteria:
Personal warmth
Communication skills with resident
Emergency responsiveness
Knowledge of dementia
Past experience working with dementia
Creativity

11. There is only seating capacity for 25 in the recreation room, but there are 30 residents who want to participate. What would you suggest doing with the additional five residents?

    Criteria:
    Initiative/Creativity
    Emergency responsiveness

12. If your judgment is questioned, how would you feel?

    Criterion:
    Receptivity to supervision

    How would you respond?

    Criterion:
    Communication skills with other staff (cohort/supervisor)

13. You discovered that a resident is missing. What would you do?

    Criteria:
    Emergency responsiveness
    Ability to work as a team

14. In the past six months, how many days have you been absent from work? (_____ Sick Days/_____ Episodes) Would you like to explain?

    Criterion:
    Attendance

15. Do you have any questions that you would like to ask me?

    Criteria:
    Communication skills with other staff (interviewer)
    Initiative

Rating Scale

Key: N/A = Not applicable
            1   = Poor
            2   = Fair
            3   = Good
            4   = Very Good
            5   = Excellent

Criteria:

1.   Personal warmth   N/A 1 2 3 4 5

2.   Communication skills with:

      residents   N/A 1 2 3 4 5

      family members   N/A 1 2 3 4 5

      other staff members   N/A 1 2 3 4 5
      (cohort/supervisor)

3.   Past experience working with:

      dementia   N/A 1 2 3 4 5

      groups   N/A 1 2 3 4 5

4.   Knowledge of dementia   N/A 1 2 3 4 5

5.   Ability to work as a team   N/A 1 2 3 4 5

6.   Initiative/creativity   N/A 1 2 3 4 5

7.   Receptivity to supervision N/A 1 2 3 4 5

8.   Emergency responsiveness N/A 1 2 3 4 5

9.   Attendance   N/A 1 2 3 4 5

                                 Total Score _____

Notes

1. Employee Rating Scale designed by Cynthia Frazier and Gail Weinstein.

2. Benenson and Teresi study at Flushing Manor and Hebrew Home for the Aged at Riverdale, New York.

3. Adapted from the curriculum of "Working With the Mentally Impaired Elderly" developed by Hunter College, City University of New York.

References

Aronson, M. K., Cox, D., Guastadisegni, P., Frazier, C., Sherlock, L., et al. (1992). Dementia and the nursing home: Associated care needs. *Journal of the American Geriatrics Society, 40,* 27-33.

Holmes, D., Teresi, U., Weiner, A., Monaco, C., Ronch, J., & Vickers, R. (1990). Impacts associated with special care units in long term care facilities. *Gerontologist, 30,* 178-183.

Knowles, M. (1969). *Higher adult education in the United States: The current picture, trend, and issues.* Washington, DC: American Council on Education.

Pines, A., Aronson, E., & Kafry, D. (1981). *Burnout: From tedium to personal growth.* New York: Free Press.

10

Legal Issues and Ethical Dilemmas in Dementia Care

Roberta S. Goodman

Joe S., a vibrant 64-year-old businessman, suffers a massive heart attack, leaving him comatose. His adult son and daughter follow the ambulance to the hospital. The emergency room physician manages to stabilize Joe S., but is now faced with deciding on a course of treatment. Joe S. cannot communicate his desires regarding medical treatment. Joe's daughter wants the hospital to do everything possible to save her father, and Joe's son does not want his father to live out his years on life support. He claims he has had many conversations with his father about quality of life issues.

Each day medical care providers and other health care professionals are confronted by ethical dilemmas. A delicate balance needs to be struck when wrestling with a decision regarding medical care for an individual who no longer has the capacity to make a decision. What should the physician do? To whom should the physician listen? What is in the best interests of the

127

patient? Is this at odds with the desires of the family? If there is
no family, who steps in for the patient?

A competent individual has the right to accept or refuse
treatment. It is when a patient's level of competency decreases
that difficulties arise in deciding to what extent that patient
may participate in determining his or her medical care. Dementia is especially difficult because the level of competency varies.

This chapter will highlight the issues that are triggered
when an incompetent individual requires medical intervention.
Who has the right to determine what treatment, if any, will be
provided? What process was used to arrive at that determination? The decisions are often complicated, particularly when
withdrawal of treatment is contemplated.

Refusal of Treatment for Incompetents: Legal Decisions

In considering the rights of incompetent patients to refuse
treatment, the Massachusetts Supreme Judicial Court, affirming
a lower court decision, reviewed *Superintendent of Belchertown v. Saikewicz*. Mr. Saikewicz was a 67-year-old severely retarded man with acute myeloblastic monocytic anemia. Weigh-
ing the likelihood of the success of known treatments (none),
the pain, and other factors, his guardian recommended to the
Court that no treatment be initiated.

The Court balanced the state's interest preserving life
against an individual's right to privacy and his right to determine treatment options. It concluded that preservation of life
does not prevail over free choice when the disease is incurable.
The Court also rejected the notion put forth in the *Quinlan*
decision in New Jersey, that courts should refrain from "gratui-
tous encroachment upon the medical profession's field of competence."

New York's position on an incompetent patient's right to
refuse care flows from two decisions—*Eichner* and *Storar.* In

the first case Brother Fox, an 83-year-old member of the Society of Mary, experienced cardiac arrest and hypoxia during routine surgery. With the aid of a respirator, he remained in a vegetative state.

When the head of the Order, Father Eichner, was informed by doctors that there was no likelihood of improvement, he requested that the respirator be removed. At trial, evidence was introduced that prior to his illness Brother Fox had made it known that he would not want extraordinary means used to prolong his life should he ever be in a hopeless vegetative state. The Court held that the right to refuse treatment is not lost as a result of incompetence and that substituted judgment would allow another person to exercise such a right on behalf of the incompetent patient.

A different decision was reached in a case involving Mr. Storar, a 52-year-old severely retarded man with a mental age of 18 months. He was diagnosed with bladder cancer. His mother was appointed his guardian and she consented to his receiving radiation treatment. After a brief remission, the disease recurred, with a diagnosis of terminal cancer. After initially consenting to transfusions, Mr. Storar's mother withdrew her consent.

The New York Court of Appeals held that the transfusions should have been continued. Unlike Brother Fox, Mr. Storar was never able to express his wishes. The Court added that if a procedural system for withdrawing treatment for incompetent patients is to be developed, the initiative should come from the legislature.

Living Wills and Health Care Proxies

In a 1988 decision, living wills were recognized by the Court of Appeals in New York as a document that could express clear and convincing evidence of a patient's wishes. Take, for example, the *Matter of O'Connor*. The majority of the Court rejected the family's wishes and granted the hospital's petition to feed the patient, a 77-year-old profoundly impaired stroke victim, through a tube. Prior to her stroke, the patient had worked in a hospital emergency room for many years. Although she had told her daughters and other persons, including nurses, that she would not want to be maintained on life support, the Court found the daughters' testimony to be "too unspecific and casual." The Court held that "the patient did not anticipate the need of a feeding tube and had made no solemn general declaration such as a living will, so there was no clear and convincing evidence of her wishes on the subject." The dissent found clear and convincing evidence of the patient's wishes, and argued that the Court should recognize some form of "substituted judgment" that could be exercised in the patient's best interests by the physician, family, or court guardian.

Living wills are accorded different weight in different jurisdictions. Although living wills can provide guidance about future medical care, they do not grant authority to anyone to make medical decisions for unanticipated situations. In 1991 the New York State legislature responded to this gap and the New York State Health Care Proxy Law became effective. Under this statute, an agent duly appointed under the proxy stands in the patient's shoes and has the legal authority to make health care decisions for the principal. Therefore, family members of nursing home residents with dementia are permitted to make medical decisions for their relatives *only* if that resident signed a health care proxy prior to becoming cognitively impaired. It should be noted that the relative power of health care proxies and living wills varies from state to state. A sample health care proxy is shown in the Appendix at the end of this chapter.

A health care facility is entitled to provide treatment, specifically, hydration and nutrition, in the absence of a specific directive from the patient to the contrary. In addition, the New York Court of Appeals held that the facility is entitled to be paid for this treatment by the person who agreed to pay for patient care upon admission (*Elbaum v. Grace Plaza of Great Neck, Inc.*, 1993).

Do Not Resuscitate Orders

Another area that has been codified and requires adherence to specific guidelines involves the Do Not Resuscitate Order (DNR). When issued, these orders are limited to resuscitation and do not relate to any other treatment. As defined by New York State Public Health Law Section 2961(4):

> Resuscitation means measures as specified in regulations promulgated by the commissioner, to restore cardiac function or to support ventilation in the event of a cardiac or respiratory arrest. Cardiac resuscitation shall *not* include measures to improve ventilation and cardiac functions in the *absence of an arrest.* (emphasis added)

An order not to resuscitate means "an order not to attempt cardiopulmonary resuscitation (CPR) in the event a patient suffers cardiac or respiratory arrest."

There is a presumption that every person consents to the administration of CPR in the event of an arrest. There is a further presumption that every person has the capacity to make a decision regarding CPR unless the attending physician determines otherwise to a reasonable degree of medical certainty or it has been determined pursuant to a court order. Even if a committee or guardian had previously been appointed, lack of capacity shall not be presumed when DNR is contemplated.

The determination of lack of capacity shall be made by the attending physician, with the concurrence of another authorized physician who personally examined the patient. Their opinion regarding the cause and nature of the incapacity, its extent, and probable duration must all be recorded in the medical chart. The patient must be informed of their findings.

A patient must consent before a DNR order can be issued, unless a discussion about CPR and the patient's condition would cause severe harm. If a finding of lack of capacity is made, a DNR order can be entered if a family member or close personal friend consents and the condition is terminal, the patient is permanently unconscious, or CPR would be medically futile or would impose an extraordinary burden in light of the condition and expected outcome of the resuscitation.

In the absence of individuals available to make this decision, DNR orders can be made in two ways. The patient's physician may issue a DNR order if CPR would be medically futile (i.e., unsuccessful in restoring cardiac or respiratory function or the patient will experience repeated arrests in a short time period before death occurs); or, a court may approve a DNR order.

A DNR order may be revoked at any time by the patient or his or her surrogate. The revocation must be immediately communicated to the physician and recorded in the patient's medical record.

When Is Substituted Judgment Triggered?

When a patient lacks the capacity to make an informed decision, a judicial process such as guardianship, committee, or conservatorship may be initiated. As defined by New York State Public Health Law, Section 2980, capacity means the ability to understand and appreciate the nature and consequences of health care decisions, including the benefits and risks thereof, and alternatives to any proposed treatment.

New York has taken a giant step closer toward respecting the unique needs of individuals with incapacities. On April 1, 1993, the legislature adopted the Mental Hygiene Law, Article 81, in response to the growing dissatisfaction with the current system of conservatorship and committee. The intent of this statute is to provide the least restrictive form of intervention to assist individuals with some incapacities to meet their needs. The guardian's powers are tailored specifically to the particular needs of a person. It was designed to afford an individual the greatest amount of independence, self-determination, and participation in all the decisions affecting a person's life. Specifically, Article 81.02(a)(1) allows the appointment of a guardian for a person "if the court determines that it is necessary to provide for the personal needs of that person, including . . . health care."

The statute does not contemplate routine diagnosis or treatment, but would allow a guardian to "consent to a medical, surgical or diagnostic intervention or procedure involving a general anesthetic which involves any significant risk or any significant invasion of bodily integrity requiring an incision or producing substantial pain, discomfort, debilitation or having a significant recovery period." The person for whom a guardian is to be appointed must agree to the appointment or be found to be incapacitated.

This statute can be a very useful vehicle for family members or a long-term care facility where medical treatment is contemplated, termination of life is not an issue, the patient is incapable of understanding the proposed treatment, much less consenting to it, and there is no health care proxy that would otherwise provide guidance and authorization. Because of its relative newness, the breadth and impact of this new and important legislation remain to be seen.

Capacity to Make Health Care Decisions

A determination that a principal lacks capacity to make health care decisions shall be made by the attending physician, to a reasonable degree of medical certainty. This finding must be documented in the patient's medical record and the patient has the right to be informed of this determination, both orally and in writing. The finding of lack of capacity becomes null and void if the patient regains capacity.

Complications arise when the proposed treatment involves hydration or nutrition. It is prohibited to withhold artificial nutrition or hydration unless the health care proxy specifically expresses the patient's desires in this regard. Absent a specific advanced directive, the agent cannot authorize termination of artificial nutrition or hydration. New York State regulations (10 NYCRR 81.1[c]) require all long-term care facilities to provide "suitable and sufficient nutrients and calories for each patient."

The Role of a Health Care Provider

New York Public Health Law Section 2991, consistent with the national Patient Self-Determination Act, which was passed in 1991, requires the facility to inform residents of their rights upon admission, to honor the directives contained in a health care proxy, and to notify the resident if the facility objects to any of the directives. In that instance, the resident has the right to be transferred to a facility that will honor the patient's decision.

The following case study painfully and eloquently demonstrates the quandary faced by health care practitioners in attempting to strike that delicate balance of individual rights versus outside influences.

Mrs. Smith, 84 years old, has been residing in a nursing home for six and a half years, over which time she has had significant cognitive decline consistent with Alzheimer's disease. After four and one-half years, her dementia necessitated her moving to a special care unit for demented individuals.

Throughout her stay, Mrs. Smith has always displayed a great sense of humor and originality and has always been considered "special" by the nursing home staff. Over the years of nursing home residence there have been only superficial, brief contacts between her and her daughter. The daughter has come to visit once or twice a year, never spending more than five minutes with her mother.

One morning about a year ago, she became ill and was diagnosed with severe congestive heart failure brought on by a total heart block—a disturbance of the conduction of electrical impulses in the heart. The physician concluded that she needed hospitalization and that implantation of a permanent pacemaker would most likely fully reverse her symptoms.

The physician called Mrs. Smith's daughter to discuss the situation and the plan of treatment. The daughter absolutely refused to consent to hospitalization and any kind of procedure such as pacemaker placement because her mother "had no life." Mrs. Smith, herself, did not have the competence to give an informed consent. The daughter had Power of Attorney for her mother's financial affairs; however, no Health Care Proxy had been executed and no agent had been appointed.

Naturally, this case led to immediate discussion between the clinical staff and the administrators. The initial decision was to manage Mrs. Smith conservatively for the next 24 hours and make a renewed effort to explain the situation to the daughter and seek her consent to the plan for treatment.

However, when the physician came to see Mrs. Smith the next morning she was not doing any better and she said, "Why do you let me lie here and die?" Upon hearing this, and despite the daughter's renewed refusal to consent, the decision was made to transfer Mrs. Smith to the hospital. At the hospital administrative consent was obtained for a pacemaker placement, despite repeated calls from the daughter's lawyer threatening to sue if the planned treatment was carried out.

The next day Mrs. Smith got her pacemaker and after a rocky course in the hospital returned to the nursing home where her recovery continued. A year later, she remains free of cardiac symptoms and is again the high spirited, albeit demented, lady who is loved by staff.

No further complaints have been received from Mrs. Smith's daughter.

This case raises many questions: Was Mrs. Smith competent to determine her medical care? Did her daughter have the legal right to object to the insertion of the pacemaker? Did the nursing home violate Mrs. Smith's rights by transferring her to a hospital? Did the nursing home violate Mrs. Smith's rights by obtaining administrative consent to have an invasive procedure performed? Whose rights prevail, Mrs. Smith's, her daughter's, or the facility's? Was the decision based on whether the treatment was in the best interests of the patient? Would Mrs. Smith have survived absent the procedure? What would her quality of life have been?

Although it is not completely clear whether Mrs. Smith was competent to make a decision regarding her medical care, she demonstrated an awareness that led her physician to conclude that his proposed course of treatment would prevail over the daughter's refusal. The scenario also suggests that Mrs. Smith's daughter did not enjoy a close relationship with her mother. She provided no details about her mother's wishes regarding what measures she would want employed or declined in the event she was not able to speak for herself. Moreover, Mrs. Smith did appoint her daughter agent over her financial matters, but did not go so far as to appoint her agent for her medical decisions. The evidence strongly supports the decision of the treating physician and the nursing home to transfer Mrs. Smith to the hospital and proceed with the surgery.

The Role of an Ethics Committee

What happens when the patient is already in an advanced state of dementia and is not competent to sign a health care proxy, much less make a decision regarding medical treatment? These complex issues, which are faced daily, are best resolved by an ethics committee staffed by the facility's medical direc-tor, director of nursing, head nurse, social service director, in-volved social worker, and an executive from administration.

The ethics committee creates a forum where differing opin-ions can be discussed and a resolution reached. Typically, the patient's treating physician is the one who has requested an opinion from the ethics committee. The physician's concerns may not be consistent with the family's. Every case is unique, and each must be considered on its own merits. The benefit of the multidisciplinary approach in staffing an ethics committee is invaluable. Each member brings professional training and education coupled with pragmatic experience. Any opinion rendered by an ethics committee is considered advisory and is not binding. It is a vehicle used to achieve a well-reasoned opinion from a group of objective individuals whose judgment is not clouded by emotion.

Quality of Life

Quality of life issues often present difficult dilemmas. Who is in the best position to judge what quality of life means? Clearly, under ideal circumstances, it is the patient. Employment of heroic measures is far more difficult to grapple with. Do you continue life support or withdraw it? Is what you do based on what the patient would have wished, or is it because of what the family wants? What if you cannot learn the patient's wishes from the patient, and substituted judgment is necessitated?

Ethics committees have become far more visible as an integral part of the decision-making process. In the absence of duly appointed agents and living wills, the burden of deciding is shared among highly qualified professionals who can assist in the judgment-making process. Health care proxies and living wills are invaluable tools in eliminating the second guessing. They provide comfort to patients who can be secure in knowing they will receive the treatment they want, or conversely, will not be subjected to treatment they would not want. They relieve the burden placed on family members, and they guide the care providers in acting legally, responsibly, and morally.

Conclusion

National statistics suggest that at least 50% of all patients in long-term care facilities have dementia. If this figure is correct, at least 700,000 persons are unable or impaired in their ability to make rational decisions about their medical treatment as a result of dementia. Many others are impaired as a result of a myriad of other conditions.

Although it is easy to write about the rules regarding advance directives and decision making or discuss them hypothetically, in reality hospitals and residential facilities daily face situations where proxies or other advance directives do not exist. Medical needs arise in patients with and without legal documentation; going to court is an extraordinary step. Practically speaking, in the absence of treatment involving a risky or painful invasive procedure or decisions contemplating termination of life, health care providers can continue to treat their patients based on what is in the patient's best interest.

Issues involved with ethical dilemmas present a far more complicated process than previously thought. After identifying the issues, the solution may still seem unattainable. To what extent can the health care provider override the family's wishes when the patient cannot speak for him- or herself? This chapter has identified legal vehicles that are available to plan for future medical care. Utilizing these tools protects those very rights. In their absence, the family and medical community must work as a unit and not hesitate to consult biomedical ethics committees. It is therefore incumbent on hospitals and nursing facilities to recognize the value of such committees and to dedicate the necessary resources to ensure that they are staffed with qualified professionals whose role is not to play god, but to help filter out the emotions and decide what is in the best interest of the patient. What becomes most apparent is that with careful planning, education, and communication many of the problematic issues presented in these hypotheticals can be avoided.

APPENDIX

Health Care Proxy

(1)   I, _____

hereby appoint _____

(name, home address, and telephone number)

_____

as my health care agent to make any and all health care decisions for me, except to the extent that I state otherwise. This proxy shall take effect when and if I become unable to make my own health care decisions.

(2)   Optional instructions: I direct my proxy to make health care decisions in accord with my wishes and limitations as stated below, or as he or she otherwise knows. (Attach additional pages, if necessary.)

_____

_____

_____

(Unless your agent knows your wishes about artificial nutrition and hydration [feeding tubes], your agent will not be allowed to make decisions about artificial nutrition and hydration. See instructions below for samples of language you could use.)

(3)   Name of substitute or fill-in proxy if the person I appoint above is unable, unwilling, or unavailable to act as my health care agent.

_____

(name, home address, and telephone number)

_____

(4)   Unless I revoke it, this proxy shall remain in effect indefinitely, or until the date or conditions stated below. This proxy shall expire (specific date or conditions, if desired):

_____

(5)   Signature _____

        Address _____

        Date _____

Statement by Witnesses (must be 18 or older)

I declare that the person who signed this document is personally known to me and appears to be of sound mind and acting of his or her own free will. He or she signed (or asked another to sign for him or her) this document in my presence.

Witness 1 _____

Address _____

Witness 2 _____

Address _____

About the Health Care Proxy

This is an important legal form. Before signing this form, you should understand the following facts:

1. This form gives the person you choose as your agent the authority to make all health care decisions for you, except to the extent you say otherwise in this form. "Health care" means any treatment, service or procedure to diagnose or treat your physical or mental condition.

2. Unless you say otherwise, your agent will be allowed to make all health care decisions for you, including decisions to remove or withhold life-sustaining treatment.

3. Unless your agent knows your wishes about artificial nutrition and hydration (nourishment and water provided by a feeding tube), he or she will not be allowed to refuse those measures for you.

4. Your agent will start making decisions for you when doctors decide that you are not able to make health care decisions for yourself.

You may write on this form any information about treatment that you do not desire and/or those treatments that you want to make sure you receive. Your agent must follow your instructions (oral and written) when making decisions for you.

If you want to give your agent written instructions, do so right on the form. For example, you could say:

If I become terminally ill, I do/don't want to receive the following treatments . . .

If I am in a coma or unconscious, with no hope of recovery, then I do/don't want . . .

If I have brain damage or a brain disease that makes me unable to recognize people or speak and there is no hope that my condition will improve, I do/don't want . . .

Examples of medical treatments about which you may wish to give your agent special instructions are listed below. This is not a complete list of treatments about which you may leave instructions.

- artificial respiration
- artificial nutrition and hydration (nourishment and water provided by feeding tube)
- cardiopulmonary resuscitation (CPR)
- antipsychotic medication
- electric shock therapy
- antibiotics
- psychosurgery
- dialysis
- transplantation
- blood transfusions
- abortion
- sterilization

Talk about choosing an agent with your family and/or close friends. You should discuss this form with a doctor or another health care professional, such as a nurse or social worker, before you sign it to make sure that you understand the types of decisions that may be made for you. You may also wish to give your doctor a signed copy. You do not need a lawyer to fill out this form.

You can choose any adult (over 18), including a family member or close friend, to be your agent. If you select a doctor as your agent, he or she may have to choose between acting as your agent or as your attending doctor; a physician cannot do both at the same time. Also, if you are a patient or resident of a hospital, nursing home or mental health facility, there are special restrictions about naming someone who works for that facility as your agent. You should ask the staff at the facility to explain those restrictions.

You should tell the person you choose that he or she will be your health care agent. You should discuss your health care wishes and this form with your agent. Be sure to give him or her a signed copy. Your agent cannot be sued for health care decisions made in good faith.

Even after you have signed this form, you have the right to make health care decisions for yourself as long as you are able to do so, and treatment cannot be given to you or stopped if you object. You can cancel the control given to your agent by telling him or her or your health care provider orally or in writing.

Filling Out the Proxy Form

Item (1) Write your name and the name, home address and telephone number of the person you are selecting as your agent.

Item (2) If you have special instructions for your agent, you should write them here. Also, if you wish to limit your agent's authority in any way, you should say so here. If you do not state any limitations, your agent will be allowed to make all health care decisions that you could have made, including the decision to consent to or refuse life-sustaining treatment.

Item (3) You may write the name, home address and telephone number of an alternate agent.

Item (4) This form will remain valid indefinitely unless you set an expiration date or condition for its expiration. This section is optional and should be filled in only if you want the health care proxy to expire.

Item (5) You must date and sign the proxy. If you are unable to sign yourself, you may direct someone else to sign in your presence. Be sure to indicate your address.

Two witnesses at least 18 years of age must sign your proxy. The person who is appointed agent or alternate agent cannot sign as a witness.

SOURCE: New York State Department of Health.

References

Elbaum v. Grace Plaza of Great Neck, Inc., 148 A.D. 244, 544 N.Y.S.2d 840, 2d Dept. (1989), rev'd. 1993, 603 N.Y.S. 2d 386.

In re Westchester County Medical Center ex. rel. O'Connor, 72 N.Y.2d 517, 534 N.Y.S. 2d 886, 531 N.E. 2d 607 (1988).

Public Health Law section 2961(17).

Matter of Eichner, 52 N.Y. 2d 363, 438 N.Y.S.2d 266 (1981), cert. den. 454 U.S. 858 (1981).

Matter of Quinlan, 355 A.2d 647, 70 N.J. 10, 79 ALR 3d 205, cert. den. 429 U.S. 922, 50 LEd 2d 289 (1976).

Matter of Storar, 52 N.Y.2d 363, 438 N.Y.S. 266 (1981), cert. den. 454 U.S. 858 (1981).

Superintendent of Belchertown State School v. Saikewicz, 370 N.E.2d 417, 373 Mass 728 (1977).

Suggested Reading

Macklin, R. (1987). *Mortal choices: Bioethics in today's world.* New York: Pantheon.

For more information, contact:

Society for the Right to Die
or
Concern for Dying Society

250 West 57th Street
New York, NY 10107

11

Reimbursement Issues and the Future Direction of Nursing Home Care for Persons With Dementia

Mary Jane Koren
Paul Guastadisegni
Miriam K. Aronson

Nursing home care is widely viewed as fiscally ruinous to individuals and government alike. Once people enter nursing homes, the average time for "spending down" to Medicaid eligibility levels is less than 6 months. From that point onward, Medicaid and, to a much lesser extent, Medicare carry the burden of paying for stays in nursing facilities.

Staff salaries account for the largest portion of nursing home costs, which have risen dramatically in recent years. Why? First, the patient population has changed markedly over the past decade. Second, expectations as to what constitutes long-term care have changed. The custodial model of care has been replaced by one in which enabling people in nursing homes to attain their highest practicable level of physical, mental, and psychosocial well-being is required.

The changing population is the result of an upward shift in age because elderly individuals are living longer. Individuals entering a nursing home fall into a spectrum of need. At one end are those admitted primarily for rehabilitative or restorative care, requiring substantial medical, professional, and allied health resources. On the other end are those still fairly physically able but cognitively impaired, requiring "high-touch" care. High-touch care requires the provision of services to meet not only physical needs but emotional, behavioral, and recreational needs. These fundamental changes—the population of older, more impaired residents and the mandate for comprehensive, individualized care—have had a substantial impact on nursing home costs in recent years. As in all other areas of health care, efforts are being made to control these costs.

Financing Long-term Care

Currently there are essentially four primary sources of payment for nursing home care: Medicare, Medicaid, long-term care insurance, and private payment.

1. *Medicare* is a federally sponsored entitlement for the elderly, linked to the Social Security system. It is targeted primarily for coverage of acute care services, whether short-term in-patient hospitalizations or intermittent, skilled services in the community. Although it covers a time-limited period of rehabilitation either in a nursing home or in a home care program, it does not cover care for individuals with ongoing supportive needs, such as individuals with dementia. Medicare pays for about 15% of nursing home days.

2. *Medicaid,* a federal/state benefits program for the medically indigent, is a needs-based program, that is, individuals

must meet stringent financial standards (regarding both income and assets) to qualify for this benefit. Because Medicaid uses state as well as federal dollars and is administered by each state, requirements vary from one state to another. Medicaid, which specifically covers nursing home stays for custodial long-term institutional and home care services, now covers over 56% of all nursing home patients on average nationally.

Both Medicare and Medicaid are supplemented by private insurance and private payment. Private insurance accounts for only about 14% of nursing home revenue and falls into two categories–Medigap and private individual insurance beyond Medigap. *Medigap* is the term used to describe a supplement to the coverage provided by Medicare in which the policy pays the copayment and deductible amounts. However, because most Medigap policies are linked to Medicare, they provide scant protection for the maintenance and supportive care services often needed by people with chronic illnesses or progressive dementias.

3. *Private long-term care insurance* is still limited in scope. Often it has been difficult to develop policies that go beyond Medigap because of erroneous beliefs by the elderly that Medicare and Medigap are sufficient, and because of denial of the actual extent of vulnerability to catastrophic long-term care expenses. Insurers have been slow to develop these policies because the benefits package is difficult to define, there is fear of expensive and open-ended liability, and there are barriers created by government regulations. Despite this, awareness is slowly coming. The purchasing power of the elderly as a group is improving and health care reform has not yet addressed nursing home payments, factors that should fuel a demand for better policies.

4. *Private payment* accounts for about 36% of nursing home revenues on average nationally, though this varies considerably from area to area and facility to facility.

Given the demographic realities and the projected need for more long-term care services, this care promises to become even more costly for society. Thus, alternative financing and cost containment are high on the political agenda.

Reimbursement

Moving from the global concerns of financing long-term care to the more specific issue of how long-term care is actually paid for in nursing homes leads to a discussion of reimbursement. In order to establish reimbursement rates that truly reflect the care provided, definitions and criteria are required. Currently there are attempts to develop a reimbursement model that will achieve this more cost effectively than previously. Historically, there was a "cost-plus" system that paid for care based on actual expenditures and thus gave incentives for increased spending, whether necessary or not. More recently, two major schemata have been proposed for reimbursement, namely a *prospective reimbursement system* and a *case-mix reimbursement system*. Both are designed to overcome the inflationary shortcoming of the cost-plus system; however, both have advantages and disadvantages.

A prospective payment system sets facility rates in advance of the payment period. This may be adjusted, however, if the rates are documented to be substantially different from actual costs. A case-mix reimbursement system, on the other hand, assesses the needs of each resident and calculates a payment rate that is a facility average, as was done in New York State. Butler (Butler & Schlenker, 1989) calls this latter a *facility-level system*. In some ways it is analogous to the type of capitation formulas used in managed care settings. It basically means that for a particular nursing home each resident receives the same level of reimbursement, based on this average, regardless of individual care requirements. This is differentiated from a *resident-level case-mix system* (Butler & Schlenker, 1989) which defines and establishes group rates. Residents are placed in hierarchical care groups that are theoretically based on physical care needs. The assignment to a case-mix category translates into the amount of reimbursement a nursing home will receive for a particular individual. A nursing home can receive several reimbursement levels under this system, as compared to the facility-level casemix system that allows one amount for every resident.

Federal Intervention: OBRA

The 1987 Omnibus Budget Reconciliation Act (OBRA) recognized the need to address reimbursement as well as quality of life and care issues because these are intertwined. OBRA recognized that a major stumbling block for the adequate reimbursement of nursing homes had been the absence of adequate assessment and systematic documentation of residents' needs. A standard instrument has emerged for the assessment of a resident's ability and capacity to function, that is, the Minimum Data Set (MDS). Most states adopted this instrument although a few created their own assessment tool to comply with OBRA. This process has become an important management issue for every nursing home, as comprehensive assessment is the cornerstone for good care planning.

Dementia Marker

Dementia is difficult to define and measure. Currently there is no specific biologic marker that can allow an accurate diagnosis and depiction of the course of an individual's dementing illness; this is, however, one area of rapid and concentrated research. Although there are several mental status screening tests in existence that can give a rough approximation of the level of cognitive impairment, they have their limitations. Mental status screens may not adequately define the remarkably different features, symptoms, abilities, and behavior problems of the residents having the same score on a test. A declining resident who can no longer communicate, resists care, is agitated, and unable to actively participate in activities, yet who maintains the physical ability and appearance of an alert, active elder differs substantially from a vegetative demented resident who can only lie in bed and vocalize simple utterances. The "alert appearing" resident is able to move freely, wander aimlessly, act out agitated behaviors, and physically resist staff, and poses a great care burden. The vegetative resident, although in a helpless state of rapid decline, is unable to offer resistance and can be routinely cared for by the nursing staff. Neither may be able to respond coherently or even comprehend the questions asked of them. The mental status test is not sensitive to different needs. The high-touch care involved with the first resident is usually overlooked in reimbursement classifications, even those employing a mental status component.

Dementia Care Requirements

Dementia is manifested by interrelated cognitive deficits, emotional and behavioral symptoms, and eventual physical dysfunction. Defining dementia care is difficult, and a single, operational definition cannot be generalized to all demented nursing home residents as patient needs fluctuate even as the disease progresses. Not all individuals with dementia manifest the same symptoms in the same way; nor is the rate of decline equal. For many residents, dementia is the precipitating cause for admission to a nursing home; for others, dementia develops after admission. Persons with dementia will, over the course of the illness, exhibit a progression of symptoms that begin as mild forgetfulness and can eventually leave the individual out of touch with the environment and self. Due to this variability of symptoms and clinical course, the diagnosis of a dementing illness in and of itself is not appropriate to determine level of care and reimbursement.

Dementia has not been identified as a cause for significant care demands and reimbursement relative to other medical conditions in most states. In New York State, for example, the assessment tool, the Patient Review Instrument (PRI)—which preceded the MDS—tended to underestimate actual care demands because the resultant reimbursement categories primarily reflected functional deficits in activities of daily living (ADL) or technology-related needs, such as oxygen, tracheostomies, catheters, and so forth, rather than the staff-intensive efforts necessary to direct, support, and guide residents with dementia. A comprehensive study of three nursing homes in New York City demonstrated that cognitive impairment *is* an important factor in determining the quantity of staff effort required by demented residents. It was also found that behavioral problems associated with cognitive decline were significantly related to perceived manageability or unmanageability of residents and that indirect care—that is, non-hands-on care—is an important component of the care of these residents (Aronson et al., 1992). Subsequently, based on data from six nursing homes, it was reported that the PRI for New York State was a significant predictor of care needs for nondemented residents. However, for demented residents the level of cognitive impairment alone was a significantly better predictor than the PRI. (Aronson, Post, & Guastadisegni, 1993).

Why Is It Difficult to Capture Care Needs?

The bottom line is that although symptoms of dementia patients can be placed on a continuum from mild to severe, variability of symptoms and behaviors, especially so-called problem behaviors, are the norm. The existence of other comorbidities, including psychiatric illness, confound the determination of what care is necessary. For example, depression is a common accompaniment to dementia, especially in mild to moderate patients, and can be responsible for "excess disability." The two must be differentiated in order to address both problems adequately.

Generally, a spectrum of interventions is required to handle the variety of behaviors associated with dementia. Although a resident without dementia is generally able to follow directions and assist in his or her care, the demented resident is generally incapable of comprehending complex directions and may resist any attempt at directed care. He or she may manifest resistance via verbal abuse, physical resistance, or refusal to participate in tasks or activities.

Behavioral Problems

Behavioral problems require that staff develop a repertoire of interventions to try to calm a resident or increase the rate of care-task completion. Success on one day does not necessarily translate into success the next time, so constant creativity is demanded of hands-on staff.

Although OBRA legislation has mandated the training of nursing aides, the amount of training specific to dementia has not been defined. Many aides lack the necessary information about, and understanding of, the nature and progression of the dementias to adequately care for demented residents.

Some demented persons retain physical ability until relatively late in the disease. They have strength and muscle movement, that is, the ability to walk, wander, push, shove, and punch, but may be incapable of reasoning out the need for walking to the bathroom or changing clothing. This can be frustrating to nursing aides who may have a patient who resists following any direction to change soiled clothes, yet who has been observed removing his or her clothing at inappropriate times during the day.

There have not been consistent findings regarding the "best" way to manage demented individuals. Because of the uneven progression of dementia and the unpredictability of its associated behavioral problems, care plans must be individualized and may require frequent revision. The need to constantly monitor these residents and modify care strategies takes staff time and effort that contribute to the costs of dementia care.

Restraint-Free Care

In the past, many nursing homes used restraints as substitutes for care, to relieve overburdened staff from the demands of mobile but difficult dementia patients, and occasionally as punishment for patients with troublesome behaviors. OBRA legislation has explicitly prohibited restraints for these purposes. One of the biggest challenges facing nursing home staff is to focus not on whether a particular device is a restraint under OBRA definitions, but rather on the etiology of the resident's behavior that caused staff to want to use a restraint. For example, staff may decide to use a seat belt or lap board to prevent a resident who has fallen from getting out of a chair because they think that the fall itself is the problem, rather than seeking underlying causes. For example, did the resident fall because the floor was wet, because his shoes didn't fit, or because of deconditioning from lack of exercise? Once the problem is approached in this way, it may become clear that the solution is not a restraint. Studies have shown that restraint reduction does not increase serious falls causing injury. In fact, it may pay dividends in improving resident well-being and staff satisfaction and in reducing costs.

Psychoactive drugs such as tranquilizers, anxiolytics, hypnotics, sedatives, and antidepressants have been overused and misused in nursing homes to restrain residents. Not only are the medications costly in and of themselves, but they also have a human cost in terms of side effects such as sleepiness, urinary retention, anorexia, Parkinsonian symptoms, and constipation. Federal law now prohibits their use unless prescribed for a specific psychiatric diagnosis and requires physicians and other staff to monitor for side effects, evidence of toxicity, and evidence of effectiveness.

Is Restraint-Free Care More Costly?

Questions have been raised as to whether restraint-free care is costlier than using restraints. Although nursing time for doing the minimum physical care required by law—that is, ambulating, turning, positioning, and documenting—may be less than when using behavioral interventions, the human toll on patients may be considerable. Patients may fall or become more agitated, incontinent and/or contracted, all of which negatively impact quality of life, and may, in fact, increase care needs and costs. The ideal would be to create a therapeutic, supportive, homelike environment that would accommodate behavioral symptoms. This may require not only design modifications of the facility but also reallocation of staff and redefinition of their roles. The dollars-and-cents impact of these changes needs further study.

New Directions for Long-Term Care

Despite the energy being expended to fix health care in general and long-term care in particular, not much headway has been achieved. Perhaps dividing the subject into four broad areas—namely, complexity, access, affordability, and quality—will make discussion somewhat easier. Clearly, these issues are interrelated; as the long-term problem is addressed they will not be able to be considered independently.

Complexity

It is common to read about the long-term care continuum, but as anyone knows who has ever tried to get a parent into a nursing home, negotiating the various agencies, programs, and paperwork quickly disabuses one of the belief in anything so straightforward. The "long-term continuum of care" is, unfortunately, one of the myths of chronic care. Chronic care is too complex to be forced into an orderly sequence of services moving in a single direction only. Reasons for this complexity abound:

- Medicaid, a joint federal/state program and the largest single payer for long-term care services, has many different ways of defining eligibility and services to be covered.
- Ideological battles rage over the "medical model" versus the "social model." Many people who need services are faced with difficulties trying to choose between programs for which there are surface distinctions without substantive differences.
- People with long-term care needs have problems that range across medical, social, physical/functional, cognitive, and psychological domains. In addition, these problems may fluctuate in severity, intensity, number, and concurrence. These characteristics mean that continual adjustments are necessary to meet client/patient needs.
- People needing long-term care include those of every economic, cultural, ethnic, and educational background. The constraints imposed by regulatory and reimbursement requirements make it difficult for any given program to adapt sufficiently to meet the needs of different subpopulations.

Access

Access to services depends on where one lives. Some states or locales simply lack programs. Even in areas apparently replete with services, access to programs may be restricted because of the eligibility criteria, which may be age-related or disability-specific, or limited by the fees charged for non-Medicaid clients.

Historically, new programs have been established with unique eligibility criteria, service constraints, and reimbursement methodology, whenever a "new" configuration of unmet needs has come to the attention of potential program sponsors. Thus, a crazy quilt of diverse services has been developed in response to short-term special interest needs rather than through a process of long-range planning.

Rather than focusing on the unique aspects of each new group, there is a need to recognize the common concerns of all groups needing long-term care and to legitimize the creative use of existing programs. AIDS is one example of the problem.

In New York City, where the number of people with AIDS made it feasible to build nursing homes, establish adult day care programs, and have special home care programs exclusively for the care of AIDS patients, the needs of this client group were well served if people were willing and able to travel to available sites. Unfortunately, it led to isolation of these individuals from the mainstream of the health care system, gave nonspecialist providers a reason to deny them access, and limited the care options available near where they lived. If, rather than focusing on the unique characteristics of the population, public efforts had gone into integrating them into existing programs and educating all providers about their needs, they would in retrospect have had more access to care.

On the other hand, this desire to be seen as unique has been fostered by the rigidity of the current health care delivery system. To a large degree it is a system in which individuals must meet the needs of programs rather than the other way around. Until existing programs are given flexibility by regulatory and reimbursement authorities to permit and encourage adaptation to evolving local demands, barriers to access will continue to plague the system.

Costs

Paying for long-term care appears to be beyond the means of individuals and government alike. For example, there are many frail, partially disabled, or demented elderly people whose families may be quite willing to provide care but who need to continue to work. Congregate day programs, which are an excellent means of providing respite for family while offering therapeutic programs for the individual, can be quite cost effective. Difficulties arise, however, because such programs tend to be rare. For example, in New York State in 1992 there were only 65 adult day health care programs; in California, only 15. Providers attempting to create such programs have sometimes found it hard to maintain a viable census. It is quite possible that the failure of Medicare or private insurance to pay for these programs for other than strictly rehabilitative purposes has made adult day health care an unavailable option for many. Eliminating day care as one of the choices offered for chronic care forces people to enter other programs, such as nursing homes or home care, both of which can be considerably more expensive.

Home care, often regarded as a panacea and a low-cost alternative to nursing home care by health planners, can quickly become a big ticket item. As people require an increasing number of hours of service, costs skyrocket. Annualized costs can run in excess of $75,000 per year for 24-hour home health aides alone, costs that do not include medications, physician visits, nursing care, medical equipment, other therapies, or even room and board. Because costs like these are rarely affordable for individuals and private policies are limited even if present, the government often is the payer of last resort. But even the deep pockets of government cannot continue to incur such staggering costs, especially as the number of people who will be needing services climbs with the age shift in the population.

Day care is also a good example of how the system has created its own dysfunction. Many communities have social model day care programs that often accommodate persons with dementia and provide the kinds of cognitive therapies and socializing activities that, while not reversing the ravages of the disease, enable patients to capitalize on residual social and intellectual functioning. Such programs are typically paid out of Title V funds and do not cover "medical services." If a person in one of these programs should have a hip fracture requiring physical therapy, he or she will need to be transferred out of the social model program and into a medical model program that may or may not be capable of continuing the dementia-specific services being received in the original program. Treating problems as discontinuous and unrelated fails to appreciate the nature of chronic illness, particularly in the elderly, and does them as well as the system a disservice both qualitatively and fiscally.

Several schemes are being tried that are breaking new ground. One, the Long-Term Care Partnership Insurance Program, a demonstration sponsored by the federal government and the Robert Wood Johnson Foundation in five states, makes insurance policies available to people up to age 84 that will provide up to 3 years of coverage in a nursing home or up to 6 years of home care (for a comparable amount of money) after which point the policyholder is automatically eligible for Medicaid without a spend-down requirement, although the usual income limits do apply. Such innovative approaches to the funding of long-term care begin to make it possible for the general public to pay for their own care without personal impoverishment or loss of hard-won assets.

Not only are ways of paying for care slowly changing but alternative sites for providing care are gradually being recognized as a further way to control costs. Options such as supportive housing, assisted living, adult foster care, and respite care are giving the chronically ill or disabled a way to maintain themselves in the least restrictive environment at much lower costs than traditional home care or nursing home care. To accomplish this, the funding streams for social support need to be integrated with those covering medically necessary care so that as individuals' needs change they can remain within a given setting and still receive appropriate services. Until the rules and regulations become flexible enough to allow the elderly and disabled to move between and among supportive and chronic care services without bureaucratic hassles, long-term care will remain a costly array of disconnected services.

Quality

The final problem that must be addressed in order to solve the long-term care problem is that of quality. Defining quality is difficult enough in acute care and ambulatory care where outcomes are quantifiable, appropriateness data is beginning to exist, and mortality rates for discrete services have been established. It is not that simple when trying to establish quality indicators in a system that must consider not only the clinical aspect of services but also the degree to which they afford recipients of that care their rights as people. Even on the purely clinical side it would be very difficult to prove that substandard medical care significantly shortened the life of a 90-year-old who had eight chronic problems, was without friends or relatives, and lived in a home without adequate plumbing. The number of variables usually encountered in a home situation may confound anyone's ability to make unequivocal judgments about the appropriateness of any single aspect of care. Further confounding attempts to improve care are ageism and therapeutic nihilism. Arguments ranging from achieving intergenerational equity to devaluing the importance of life to a disabled individual make raising standards a Herculean task.

Because of the losses, both tangible and intangible, which accompany living in a nursing home, and because of the poor quality of life in many facilities, many older people say they would prefer death to nursing home admission. Whether the newest fad for improving quality, total quality management, is able to succeed where internal quality assurance committees and external surveying and accrediting bodies have failed remains to be seen. However, until the providers of long-term care, particularly institutional care, take a hard look at their current practices and create programs and services that are more user-friendly, the future of long-term care may well be a dim one.

The need for long-term care will always exist, and meaningful solutions must be developed. An important first step is to conceptualize a long-term care system that is not modeled as a continuum. This new system must be organized to take into account the way people's lives and their medical and psychosocial conditions are linked, so that what they need is available when they need it, in a way that respects their dignity and protects their rights. In addition, the responsibility of paying for care must be shared between the recipients of that care and the government in a way that bankrupts neither. Accomplishing this will truly be the challenge of the 21st century because it is highly unlikely that the problem of long-term care is yet acute enough to force the needed changes.

References

Aronson, M. K., Cox, D., Guastadisegni, P., Frazier, C., Sherlock, L., Grower, R., Barbera, A., Sternberg, M., Breed, J., & Koren, M. J. (1992). Dementia and the nursing home: Association with care needs. *Journal of the American Geriatrics Society, 40,* 27-33.

Aronson, M. K., Post, D. C., & Guastadisegni, P. (1993). Dementia, agitation, and care in the nursing home. *Journal of the American Geriatrics Society, 41,* 507-512.

Butler, P. A. & Schlenker, R. E. (1989). Case-mix reimbursement for nursing home payment: Resource utilization groups, Version II. *Health care financing review supplement,* 39-52.

Suggested Readings

Alzheimer's Disease and Related Disorders Association. (1992). *"Don't count on it!": A report on long-term care insurance coverage of Alzheimer's disease.* Chicago: Author.

Alzheimer's Disease and Related Disorders Association. (1992). *A legal and financial planning guide for New Yorkers: A report on the fiscal and legal resources for families coping with Alzheimer's disease.* Chicago: Author.

Buchanan, R. J., Madel, R. P., & Persons, D. (1991). Medicaid payment policies for nursing homes: Objectives and achievements. *The Milbank Quarterly, 67,* 103-136.

Butler, P. A., & Schlenker, R. E. (1989). Case-mix reimbursement for nursing home payment: Resource utilization groups, Version II. *Health Care Financing Review,* Suppl., 39-52.

Glossary

Activities of daily living (ADL). Those functions such as bathing, dressing, toileting, ambulating, and eating that are part of daily routine. Functional ability is measured by ability to perform ADL tasks.

Advance directives. An advanced directive enables an individual to control decisions about health care in the event he or she becomes unable to make his or her own decisions in the future. The advance directive may be a health care proxy, a living will, or a combination of both. The advance directive may be used to accept or to refuse any treatment or procedure used to diagnose, treat, or care for any physical or mental condition, including life-sustaining treatment.

Assisted living. A broad spectrum of residential options for the frail elderly including foster care, board and care, residential care, boarding homes, and congregate living. These facilities have available a range of services including supervision, personal care, and nursing, and can often be viable alternatives to nursing home care.

Burnout. A problem commonly ascribed to health care workers, many of whom work under stressful conditions.

Capacity. The ability to understand and appreciate the nature and consequences of health care decisions, including the benefits, risks, and alternative to any proposed treatment, and to be able to reach an informed decision.

Case-mix reimbursement system. A form of long-term care reimbursement whereby the amount is determined by the acuity of the residents. Two forms of reimbursement fall under this category, both based on an average. In one instance the average is drawn from the entire nursing home population, combining both extremes of the care continuum, and an overall reimbursement rate, which is exactly the same for each resident, is derived. The second method places individuals in particular categories based on their care needs and provides a separate reimbursement rate for each category.

Catastrophic reaction. Overreaction by individuals with therapeutic stimuli or situations that do not warrant these behaviors. These reactions are often unpredictable.

Chemical restraints. A pharmaceutical given with the sole purpose of inhibiting or controlling resident behavior or altering mood or mind. These include sedatives, psychotropics (such as tranquilizers and antipsychotic medications), and antihistamines (which are sometimes used solely for their sedating side effects).

Cognitive stimulation. The use of verbal and/or nonverbal activities to maximize existing abilities and increase sensory awareness.

Competency. Any adult over the age of 18 years is presumed competent. This is a legal term used to describe a person's ability to make informed choices, such as regarding a contract, a will, or a health care decision.

Cuing. An intervention in which a staff member provides enough prompts so that an individual may do as much as possible for himself or herself, rather than doing actual hands-on care.

Delirium. An acute mental disorder characterized by decreased awareness of the surrounding environment and fluctuating ability to maintain proper attention to people and objects nearby.

Dementia. A decline in memory and other intellectual functions in an alert individual and associated declines in functional abilities and behavior. Dementia may be caused by a number of conditions, of which Alzheimer's disease is the most common.

Dementia care units. Dementia-specific special care units are based on the concept of homogeneous groupings of patients and generally target activities and staffing for ambulatory confused and agitated residents.

Depression. A psychiatric syndrome whose symptoms may include persistently low mood with lack of interest, low energy, loss of appetite, change in sleep pattern, and feelings of worthlessness and/or hopelessness. Symptoms of dementia and depression overlap and these two conditions may occur concurrently.

Do not resuscitate order (DNR). A DNR means an order not to attempt cardiopulmonary resuscitation (CPR) in the event a patient suffers cardiac or respiratory arrest. Resuscitation means measures to restore cardiac function or to support ventilation in the event of a cardiac or respiratory arrest. It does not include measures to improve ventilation and cardiac functions in the *absence* of an arrest.

Health care proxy. A legal document that appoints an individual (agent) who will make health care decisions for the preparer when that individual lacks the capacity to do so for him- or herself. In some states, a health care proxy may replace a living will. In others, it is necessary to have both documents.

Iatrogenic costs. Costs that are created by medical interventions, that is, adverse reactions from medications, complications of surgery, restraints, and so forth.

Informed consent. Consent given only after the patient has been apprised of the nature, risks, benefits, and alternatives to a proposed medical treatment or research study.

In-house day care. An activities-based program for nursing home residents, whereby the residents leave their units for a program of socialization, activities, and meals. In addition to the benefits for residents, unit staff and other residents get needed respite when the more difficult residents are in the program.

Least restrictive environment. The use of alternative strategies to manage behaviors that would otherwise be problems and might trigger restraint use. For example, when residents wander, it is preferable to provide a secured "wandering path" for them rather than to use physical or chemical restraints. The least restrictive measures that would not jeopardize the resident's safety should be used before more restrictive measures.

Living will. A document that expresses a patient's wishes regarding future medical care. The relative power of health care proxies and living wills vary from state to state.

Long-term care insurance. Privately purchased insurance to help cover the expense of home care and nursing home costs. A viable policy should include the following: (a) access to insurance for Alzheimer's patients; (b) coverage of care requirements related to cognitive impairment; (c) payment for home and community care; (d) payment for alternative residential care; (e) lapse protection, to ensure that persons with cognitive impairment who fail to make a policy payment as a direct result of their impairment can have their coverage maintained; and (f) inflation protection, to ensure the value of the policy is sufficient to maintain its viability regardless of changes in the economic situation of society. (Taken from a report by the Alzheimer's Association on long-term care insurance, 1992.)

Medicaid. A program funded by both federal and state governments to provide health services for low-income individuals of all ages, as well as for those who have exhausted their financial resources or insurance (medically indigent). Medicaid pays for a significant proportion of long-term care costs.

Medicare. A federally funded health insurance for the aged and disabled that is connected with the Social Security system and is primarily involved in providing coverage for acute care. This insurance does not cover the cost of custodial long-term care services in an individual's home or in a nursing home.

Nonverbal communication. The process of transmitting and receiving information with facial expressions, body language, posture, and other means.

Omnibus Budget Reconciliation Act of 1987 (OBRA). The legislation that embodies the provisions for nursing home reform (Public Law 100-203).

Patient Self-Determination Act. A federal law that requires hospitals and nursing homes to advise patients on admission of the applicable state laws regarding living wills and health care proxies and their rights regarding advance directives.

Physical restraints. Any physical or manual device, material, or equipment attached or adjacent to the resident's body that the individual cannot remove easily that restricts freedom of movement or normal access to one's body. These include camisoles or vests, ankle and wrist appliances, geriatric chairs (with lapboards), bedside rails (under specific circumstances, may vary by state), locked doors, belts, and harnesses.

Problem solving. Alzheimer care requires dealing with unpredictable behaviors and situations. Interventions often involve the team members' brainstorming to devise strategies for solution of these problems.

Prospective payment system. A system of reimbursement that sets facility rates in advance of the payment period.

Quality of life. The current level of an individual's comfort and enjoyment.

Reminiscence. An activity used to assist in the cognitive stimulation process by emphasizing one's past experiences and memories and association of these recollections to elicit a verbal or nonverbal response.

Restraint monitoring. When physical restraints are used, they should be released as frequently as necessary to meet individual resident care needs for toileting, exercise, and so forth, but at least every 2 hours except when the resident is in bed asleep. Restrained residents must also be observed at the time of dressing and undressing for any evidence of adverse effects, including but not limited to circulatory problems or skin abrasions. In addition, the facilitywide frequency, type of restraints, and trends in use should be monitored as part of the facility's quality assurance program.

Role change. On admission, family caregivers must relinquish their responsibility for their loved one's physical care yet remain involved in the caring as a member of the caregiving team.

"Spending down." Medicaid eligibility has strict income and asset requirements. Individuals with limited means who require Medicaid assistance for health services must use their resources before they are eligible, that is, they must spend down to meet criteria.

Substituted judgment. The designated decision maker must stand in the patient's shoes, considering what the patient would have wanted had he or she been able to render a decision regarding a proposed course of medical care.

Sundowning. A dementia-associated phenomenon whereby the level of confusion and associated agitation seem to increase markedly in the late afternoon or early evening.

Support group. Group meetings are held for patients and/or family members to receive information and emotional support regarding a common disease or problem. In many facilities, these group meetings are held for family members to help them cope with the institutionalization of a loved one.

Task segmentation. A type of assistance for individuals with dementia in which an activity is divided into single steps or tasks that can be completed by the patient one at a time.

Team approach. Dementia care requires efforts of caregivers from multiple disciplines, including nursing, medicine, social work, activities, other therapies, and interested family members, working collaboratively as a team.

Therapeutic nihilism. An attitude that treatment is not worth the effort. Although this may occur regarding people of any age, it is more prevalent regarding the elderly. This may be a form of ageism, whereby individuals equate aging and illness.

Index

About the Authors

Miriam K. Aronson, Ed.D., is Director of the Institute on Aging at Bergen Pines County Hospital, Paramus, NJ, and is an Associate Professor of Epidemiology and Social Medicine and Psychiatry at the Albert Einstein College of Medicine. She was the founding chair of the Education and Public Awareness Committee of the National Alzheimer's Association, has been editor of the Alzheimer's Association Newsletter for 7 years, and has served as an educational consultant for several years. A licensed nursing home administrator, she has been on several New York City, New York state, and national advisory groups regarding Alzheimer's care, long-term care and health care financing. Her major research interests are the oldest old and the development of dementia. Dr. Aronson has authored and coauthored many peer-reviewed publications in professional journals, has been a contributor to several books, and has edited two books, including *Understanding Alzheimer's Disease* (1988). She has given more than 200 presentations nationally and internationally. She received her doctorate in social gerontology from Teacher's College, Columbia University.

Leonard Berg, M.D., is Professor of Neurology and Director of the Alzheimer's Disease Research Center at Washington University. He is a member of the Alzheimer's Association's Board of

174

Directors and is chair of its Medical and Scientific Advisory Board. His research efforts have focused on diagnostic criteria and natural history studies in Alzheimer's disease (AD) and on the distinction between mild AD and "normal aging," especially in the very old. He is Chair of the Advisory Panel of the National Institute on Aging (NIA) Collaborative Studies on Dementia Special Care Units and is advisor to several of the NIA-funded Alzheimer's Disease Centers across the country. For eight years he was Director of the American Board of Psychiatry and Neurology (ABPN), including one year as its President.

Randi C. Dressel, B.A., is the Chief Operating Officer of Menorah Campus, Inc. She holds a B.A. in Interdisciplinary Studies with a major in gerontology from the State University of New York at Buffalo. She has been working in the field of gerontology since 1975.

David M. Dunkelman, M.S., J.D., is President of Menorah Campus, Inc., a community-based continuum of care in Western New York. He holds an M.S. in Long-Term Care Administration from the University of North Texas, Denton, Texas, and a law degree from Temple University, Philadelphia, PA.

Cynthia Frazier, Ph.D., is a clinical psychologist currently in private practice in Carmel, New York. She specializes in the treatment of the elderly. As Director of Mental Health at Sea View Hospital and Home in Staten Island, New York, she developed one of the first dementia units for the elderly. Later, as Director of Clinical Programs and Education at Morningside House Nursing Home, she implemented several programs for the demented including SHARE, an in-house day care program. She has taught at the university level, presented lectures and workshops nationally and internationally, and published several clinical papers and book chapters.

Patricia Gaston, A.C.S.W., is the Director of Dementia Care Services at The Home for Aged Blind in Yonkers, NY. The facility has a 22-bed special care unit for mild to moderately ambulatory, visually impaired dementia residents. Ms. Gaston has been involved in its operation and management since its inception in 1988. She has been an active family support group leader for the local Alzheimer's Association over the past several years and has participated in research on Alzheimer's Disease. She has coauthored several publications and has presented at numerous conferences.

Roberta S. Goodman, Esq., J.D., is an attorney who practices in Irvington, New York. She is the immediate past president of the New York City Chapter of the Alzheimer's Association.

Helene D. Grossman, M.S., L.N.H.A., has been the Associate Executive Director of Hebrew Home for the Aged at Riverdale and Vice President, Director of J.G.B. Health Facilities Corp., an affiliate of the Jewish Guild for the Blind. Her extensive experience in the field of aging includes the management and long-term care and housing facilities, adult day health care and other out-patient services. She has published and lectured on such subjects as dementia care services, quality of life, resident empowerment, congregate housing, and other aspects of long-term care managemment.

Ronnie Grower, M.A., has been a researcher and consultant in the fields of gerontology and health care for the past 20 years. Her work includes studies on in-house day care programs for Alzheimer's patients; the needs of nursing home residents with dementia; the use and misuse of medications among the elderly; hospice; health promotion services for the young elderly; and the effectiveness of employment programs for mature SSDI beneficiaries. She is Director of Utilization Management for Sierra Health Services in Las Vegas, Nevada, and is a research consultant for Aging in America. She has master's degrees from Pennsylvania State University and Teacher's College, Columbia University.

Paul Guastadisegni, M.A., is a doctoral candidate in Health Psychology at the Albert Einstein College of Medicine/Ferkauf Graduate School of Psychology. He is a research assistant at Columbia Psychiatric Institute.

Mary Jane Koren, M.D., began her career in geriatrics at Montefiore Medical Center and the Albert Einstein School of Medicine. Later, as the Director of Long Term Care Services at the New York State Department of Health she took the lead on implementing OBRA 87 in New York. Currently she is in charge of the health care quality improvement initiative, part of the new PRO program to use data analysis to profile provider practices and patient outcomes. She teaches Health Policy Analysis at New York University and is conducting several health services research projects in long-term care.

Patricia Krasnausky, L.N.H.A., has more than 20 years of health care management and consulting experience. She is a licensed Nursing Home Administrator and is currently the Administrator of Cabrini Nursing Home in New York City. She was the Administrator of Frances Schervier Home & Hospital during the Restraint Release Demonstration Program.

Karen J. Lazar, M.A., is a doctoral candidate in Health Psychology at the Albert Einstein College of Medicine/Ferkauf Graduate School of Psychology. She is also an analyst-in-training at the Psychoanalytic Center of Northern New Jersey, and a research fellow at Bergen Pines Institute on Aging in Paramus, NJ.

Susan Leventer, Ph.D., is Director of Rehabilitation at the Jewish Home of Rochester in Rochester, New York. She received her master's degree in Speech Pathology-Audiology from the State University of New York at Genesee and a Ph.D. degree in Psychology from the University of Rochester. Her research, publications, and presentations have emphasized the importance of language and cognitive factors in rehabilitation. She was principal investigator for the NYS Health Department grant to encourage innovation in long-term care at Kirkhaven, a not-for-profit facility in Rochester, NY.

Deborah Lynch, M.S.N., has been Director of Nursing at Frances Schervier Home and Hospital since 1986. She has wide experience in geriatric care, especially with dementia patients. In 1989 she was Project Director for the facility's Restraint-Reduction Demonstration Program funded by a grant from the

New York State Department of Health. She was instrumental in expanding the restraint-reduction program throughout the facility. She is coauthor of "Harnessing Ideas to Release Restraints," in *Geriatric Nursing,* May/June 1991. She is a licensed registered nurse in Pennsylvania and New York. She received an M.A. degree in Social Gerontology and an M.S. in Gerontological Nursing, both from the University of Pennsylvania.

Theresa Martico-Greenfield, M.P.H., L.N.H.A., is the Assistant Administrator at The Jewish Home and Hospital for Aged, Manhattan Division. She has published and spoken on topics relating to bioethics, community services, and institutional long-term care. She has taught at New York University and Columbia University and is an active participant in professional associations including the American Society on Aging.

Donna Cox Post, Ph.D., received her doctorate in developmental psychology from SUNY Stony Brook, and since 1987 has been involved in nursing home research with her work at the Brookdale Center on Aging. Her association with Dr. Aronson began in 1989 when she became project coordinator for a study funded by the Alzheimer's Initiative of the New York State Department of Health. The purpose of the project was to examine the adequacy of nursing home reimbursement in relation to the care needs of cognitively impaired residents. Dr. Post currently is a member of the Research Department of the National League for Nursing, where she is working on examination of trends in nursing education and the supply and demand for nurses in the workforce, especially with regard to health care reform policies.

Barry Rovner, M.D., is an Associate Professor in the Department of Psychiatry and Human Behavior at Jefferson Medical College, and Medical Director of the Geriatric Psychiatry Unit at Wills Eye Hospital, Philadelphia, PA. Prior to joining the staff at Jefferson in 1991, he was Associate Professor at Johns Hopkins University in Baltimore, and was medical director and consultant for Alzheimer's units in nursing homes. He received an NIMH award for "A Randomized Trial of Dementia Care

in Nursing Homes" to develop a ⸝
demented nursing home patients. ⸝
Medical College, and was a resident ⸜
in neuropsychiatry at Johns Hopkins Uᵢ.
cine. He has written and spoken extensivε.   179
and treatment of dementia in the elderly.

ᵢ *in*

Lila Sherlock, R.N., C., M.S.N., is a nurse pracᵢ
Geriatric Division of Montefiore Medical Center iᵢ.
and Geriatric Nursing Educator at the Margaret Tietz ᶜ
Nursing Care in Queens, N.Y. She received her undergᵢ
nursing degree from Hunter-Bellevue and an M.S.in nuᵢ
from Columbia University. She has experience in care of the
elderly in hospital, community and nursing home settings.
Since 1983, she has been involved in research in dementia and
aging, and with grant support from the Commonwealth Fund
and the United Way, has helped develop programs to train
nursing home staff to care for dementia patients.

Cynthia Wallace, R.N., M.A., has been in the long-term care
field for 20 years. She is currently Executive Vice President and
was formerly CEO of Morningside House Nursing Home Com-
pany, Inc. She has lectured, conducted numerous workshops,
and served on state and national committees dealing with
long-term health care. She is a member of the Board of Directors
of the New York Association of Homes and Services for the
Aging (NYAHSA) and chairs the NYAHSA Nursing Facility Sub-
Committee and the Education and Research Committee.

Gail Weinstein, M.S., L.N.H.A., is a licensed Nursing Home
Administrator and is Vice President for Clinical Programs and
Public Relations for Morningside House, Aging in America and
United Presbyterian Residence. She oversees the operation of
the Corporation's three Alzheimer's Adult Day Health Care Programs. She was responsible for the creation, development and
implementation of these programs, as well as for Morningside's
Long Term Home Health Care Program and an in-house day care
program in the nursing home for residents with dementia.